Plagues,
Products,
and Politics

Plagues, Products, and Politics

Emergent Public Health Hazards and National Policymaking

Christopher H. Foreman, Jr.

The Brookings Institution
WASHINGTON, D.C.

Copyright © 1994 by
THE BROOKINGS INSTITUTION
1775 Massachusetts Avenue, N.W., Washington, D.C. 20036

Library of Congress Cataloging-in-Publication data

Foreman, Christopher H.
  Plagues, products, and politics : emergent public health
hazards and national policymaking / Christopher H.
Foreman.
    p.   cm.
  Includes bibliographical references and index.
  ISBN 0-8157-2876-X (cloth)—ISBN 0-8157-2875-1
    1. Health risk assessment—Government policy—
United States.   2. Crisis management in government—
United States.   3. Medicine, Preventive—Government
policy—United States.   4. Product safety—Government
policy—United States.   5. Epidemics—United States.
6. AIDS (Disease)—Government policy—United States.
I. Title.
  RA394.F67   1994
  614.4'0973—dc20   94-15189
                                                            CIP

9 8 7 6 5 4 3 2 1

The paper used in this publication meets the minimum
requirements of the American National Standard for Information Sciences—Permanence of paper for Printed Library
Materials, ANSI Z39.48—1984

Typeset in Palatino

Composition by INNODATA Publishing Services Division
Hanover, Maryland

Printed by R. R. Donnelley and Sons Co.
Harrisonburg, Virginia

Foreword

The American public fears for its health in many ways. Chronic threats such as cancer and heart disease are a familiar worry. Another concern, however, is the infectious disease or dangerous product that victimizes quickly and perhaps in ways unfamiliar to the general public. Although science, sanitation, and regulation have triumphed over diseases such as polio and smallpox and ended the most egregious horrors of product adulteration, new or suddenly prominent dangers, whether natural (AIDS, Lyme disease) or artificial (hazardous medical devices), still pose significant policy challenges.

In this volume Christopher H. Foreman, Jr., a senior fellow in the Brookings Governmental Studies program, offers a wide-ranging discussion of emergent public health hazards. Despite public expectation that the federal government will handle health and safety problems swiftly and effectively, he argues, the appropriate agencies remain largely hostage to technical uncertainties and external political forces that are often hard to overcome. Although critics often point their finger at an agency's upper echelons, Foreman shows how policy tends to be shaped more often by technical and political constraints than by the quality or commitment of agency leadership. Foreman advocates improved national and global surveillance as an essential and politically feasible weapon against emergent public health hazards.

The author wishes to thank several persons who read all or part of the manuscript. They include Christopher J. Bosso, Stephen Klaidman, Thomas E. Mann, Gilbert S. Omenn, Paul J. Quirk, Bert A. Rockman, Harvey M. Sapolsky, R. Kent Weaver, Joseph White, and James Q. Wilson. He also appreciates the helpful discussions with Mark C. Rom, formerly at the General Accounting Office. Daniel A. Hofherr, Lawrence F. Jindra, Paul Joyce, Jonathan Kay, Mark Lotwis, and Ilyse Veron offered research assistance at various stages of this project.

At Brookings, Colleen McGuiness edited the manuscript, Alison Rimsky and Eric Messick verified it, and Susan Woollen prepared it for typesetting. Rhonda Holland constructed the index, and Ingeborg Lockwood and Cynthia Terrels assisted in the preparation of the manuscript.

The views expressed here are solely those of the author and should not be ascribed to the persons whose assistance is acknowledged above or to the trustees, officers, or other staff members of the Brookings Institution.

BRUCE K. MACLAURY
President

July 1994
Washington, D.C.

Contents

One

Visible Victims

T HIS BOOK is about unpleasant surprises. It examines the American national government's capacity to respond to a diverse but distinctive category of public health problem: the suddenly prominent, and often newly recognized, imminent hazard that may spread unless contained. The threats discussed include communicable diseases such as acquired immunodeficiency syndrome (AIDS), Lyme disease, Legionnaires' disease, and drug-resistant tuberculosis (TB) as well as product-related dangers such as injurious vaccines, silicone breast implants, and cyanide-laced Tylenol. These problems share traits that make prompt and effective action desirable but differ dramatically in their susceptibility to intervention.[1] Because such hazards can cause serious harm to identifiable individuals and could victimize more widely unless something is done, aggressive federal involvement usually is expected.

What can the national government realistically deliver? Government's responsibility is to investigate the scope, severity, and cause of victimization. If the problem is a product, regulators might want to withdraw it or limit its availability. Government may also facilitate the search for, or distribution of, ameliorative technologies and preventive information. The environment in which government must do all these things imposes many constraints. The most basic and crucial one is the state of relevant technical knowledge and how easy it is to acquire. But institutional and political factors also hinder effectiveness. Bureaucrats, politicians, and organized interests may disagree among themselves. Federal officials may also be unable to influence adequately state-level and local dynamics, and public health is predominantly a state and local function. An independent media may be an engine of excessive fear or an invaluable tool for public education and awareness. Agencies

1

at all levels may have to reallocate resources or reorganize to handle a new problem. The way society at-large regards hazard victims, and whether those victims are vocal or silent, is also significant.

The dangers discussed here confront federal policymakers with at least five broad and overlapping tasks: outbreak discovery; field investigation; field intervention (including education for professionals and the public); the regulation of products and processes; and biomedical research. This book examines the blend of technical, institutional, and political challenges inherent in these tasks. Each produces different constraints from every other (even for the same hazard), and success is often limited, underappreciated, or difficult to evaluate.

Two overlapping tensions afflict policymaking for emergent public health hazards. The first is the challenge of striking a workable and justifiable balance between urgency and restraint. The practical difficulty of striking such a balance in public health is formidable and in some respects resembles the formulation of national defense policy. When confronted by a resourceful and unpredictable military foe, the nation might have to be rallied quickly in support of tangible countermeasures while remaining sensitive to limited knowledge, shifting circumstances, and the possibility that some types of response might either make war more likely or strengthen the enemy's hand should war break out. On the one hand, a state of continued alert may be hard to sustain and may prove costly, in ways both tangible and intangible, if substantial resources are committed but no major threat emerges. No one wants a disruptive panic. On the other hand, tardy response is also intolerable. Failure to anticipate or to respond quickly to a significant threat invites blame. Neither public health officials nor military commanders want to have to explain to administrative superiors, politicians, or inquiring reporters why caution prevailed when vigorous action was clearly called for.

The AIDS epidemic has become the most complex balancing act between urgency and restraint in public health. Health authorities and AIDS activists tell the American people to view AIDS as a grave and immediate threat, but not to succumb to panic or encroach on the rights of infected persons. Efforts to straddle the divide between urgency and restraint risk confusing the public, however. As one perceptive journalist observed in mid-1991:

Having told the public for years that AIDS was such a threat that it demanded changes in fundamental human behavior, many [researchers and public health officials] wonder whether it is now too late to turn around and tell the world that AIDS poses no special risk in the health care setting or from immigrants. And if AIDS really does become like just any other disease, how will it be possible to maintain its privileged political status as the medical condition on which more is spent per capita than any other in U.S. history?[2]

The second tension is the extent to which decisionmaking by scientific or technical experts can and should be insulated from politics.[3] The word *politics* carries at least two connotations. One is anchored in self-interest. Individuals and institutions try to maximize credit, avoid blame, conserve power, and protect their interests.[4] For scientists and officials alike, *political* often implies "undesirably nonscientific." More broadly, the term describes the struggle to govern—the process by which agendas emerge, coalitions form or expire, and fundamental public values (accountability, fairness, responsiveness, and efficiency) claim attention.[5]

Every aspect of the way society handles hazards to human health is inherently political in both senses. Once victimization by disease has occurred, the problem must be both recognized and believed worth reacting to. Enlarging the share of staff time, research funds, or regulatory enforcement committed to a problem requires that its priority be raised where it counts—in the relevant government agencies and, in some cases, among elected officials and the general public. And the resulting agendas and policies are never fixed but are instead continually open to challenge and renegotiation. After more than a decade and many tens of thousands of deaths in the United States alone, the priority given to the AIDS epidemic is still contested. Some activists remain convinced that the government is not doing enough, despite the thorough institutionalization of the disease as a top priority among public health agencies and the evolution of a virtual "AIDS establishment."[6] Meanwhile, some critics argue that the epidemic has been oversold, displacing attention and draining resources that could be better deployed elsewhere.[7] Other ailments such as Lyme disease and chronic fatigue syndrome engage smaller and less aggressive constituencies and are less visible to politicians, but they are political in the same sense.

Though essential, the political process tends to be messy and unpredictable. The behavior of journalists, organized interests, and politicians may have both positive and negative effects. Their attention may generate additional resources, heightened accountability, and necessary public awareness. But a perception of crisis or insufficient response might also spawn destructive political meddling, stressful (and perhaps unnecessary) change in established agency routines or priorities, and undue public alarm. Controversy is hard to anticipate or control once unleashed. Organized interests will push for either a more aggressive response or a more restrained one, independently of (and perhaps in opposition to) the desires of government officials.

Professed dissatisfaction among even successful policy advocates is not surprising and must be interpreted with caution. Advocates succeed, in part, by asserting that their efforts have borne insufficient fruit. Such claims, a routine part of the political process, keep followers and allies mobilized, the press attentive, and target institutions on the defensive. Advocates are cross-pressured to appear both reasonable and tough, with the relative emphasis depending on the circumstances. Moreover, only something close to a genuine state of war (not the occasional bursts of attention to ongoing problems such as poverty, cancer, or illegal drugs that sponsors hyperbolically trumpet as war) elicits from the nation the kind of coordinated and committed emergency response that would satisfy advocates.

Public policies generally should be effective and balanced, maximizing positive impact while minimizing damaging diversions and various kinds of overkill. Health hazards are no exception. The central theme of this volume is that government's ability to achieve ideal public policy hinges mostly on characteristics and uncertainties inherent in specific hazards, and on conflicts uncontrollably provoked by them, far more than on the strategies and leadership of federal agencies. This book does not posit, let alone specify, a precise path to the perfect balancing of the tensions it demonstrates. But a review of past problems can be useful for coping with future ones despite the unpredictability of hazards yet to come. History can be instructive and, among other things, teaches its students to be wary of refighting the same wars.

A Litany of Problems

At the beginning of the 1980s a general impression existed that the battle against infectious diseases had been largely won in the industrialized Western nations. The result was a complacency later widely recognized as misguided.[8] With smallpox officially proclaimed eradicated, and many other communicable scourges largely tamed by the combined assaults of science and sanitation, an era of chronic and degenerative ailments seemed to have dawned.[9] A much-noted irony is that the most feared and publicized health threat of the 1980s would turn out to be an infectious disease: AIDS triggered by the spread of the human immunodeficiency virus (HIV).[10] Since the early 1970s numerous other public health threats posing serious and quickly manifested harm achieved sudden, and usually brief, prominence:

—In 1976 Americans were told by the federal government that a particularly virulent strain of influenza, the so-called swine flu, might soon appear, perhaps to cause a degree of flu-associated illness and death not seen since the infamous 1918–19 pandemic that killed more than half a million persons in the United States alone.[11]

—In the summer of 1976 a previously unknown ailment struck 182 persons attending the Pennsylvania state convention of the American Legion. Of these, 29 would die.[12] Ever since, Legionnaires' disease has been part of the lexicon of public health, and outbreaks recur.[13]

—In late 1976 the swine flu vaccine program was abruptly halted when officials discovered an association between the vaccine and a rare ascending paralysis called Guillain-Barré syndrome (GBS). Although swine influenza did not sweep the United States, 532 vaccinees would contract GBS, leading to 32 deaths.[14]

—In the early 1980s American women learned that tampons used to absorb menstrual flow could also produce a serious and potentially deadly condition called toxic shock syndrome (TSS). Although an average of 420 cases of TSS per year was reported to the Centers for Disease Control (CDC) during the period 1983–88, the actual number of cases was doubtless much higher.[15]

—In the early 1970s an intrauterine contraceptive device used by more than 2 million American women, the Dalkon Shield, caused painful infections and irrevocable injuries, including infertility, triggering litigation that would stretch throughout the 1980s.[16]

—In the 1980s Reye's syndrome (RS), a rare and sometimes fatal condition striking children after they took aspirin for flu or chicken pox, captured headlines across the country. The number of cases reported to the CDC reached a high of 555 in 1980, declining to a mere 20 by 1988 because adults had learned to avoid giving aspirin to ill children. As with TSS, the peak figure for reported cases understated the true incidence of RS.[17]

—In 1979 two soy-based infant formulas, inadvertently rendered chloride-deficient, were found to cause serious metabolic disturbances, prompting a recall, a wave of publicity, and a congressional investigation resulting in new protective legislation. In 1982 a batch of vitamin-deficient formula triggered another public scandal.[18]

—In the autumn of 1982, the nation was stunned by reports that capsules of Tylenol, a popular pain-reliever, had been emptied, refilled with cyanide, and placed back on a store shelf in the Chicago area. Seven persons died as a result. In February 1986 a woman in Yonkers, New York, died when she, too, took cyanide masquerading as Tylenol, causing another wave of media attention and public concern.[19]

—In 1984 an intravenous form of vitamin E known as E-Ferol, marketed without Food and Drug Administration (FDA) approval, was implicated in thirty-eight infant deaths, prompting a congressional investigation.[20]

—In 1988 the United States reported some five thousand cases of Lyme disease, an ailment first recognized in the mid-1970s and associated with headache, fever, arthritic symptoms—it was originally dubbed Lyme arthritis—and neurological abnormalities.[21]

—In late 1989 public health authorities reported that an over-the-counter diet supplement, L-tryptophan, was associated with a rare blood disorder called eosinophilia-myalgia syndrome. L-tryptophan was recalled, but not before thousands had been poisoned and twenty-seven were killed by what turned out to be a contaminant.[22]

—Beginning in the early 1980s large numbers of persons, young Caucasian women in particular, began to seek treatment for what public health authorities would ultimately label chronic fatigue syndrome (CFS). An ailment whose onset is often marked by flu-like symptoms, CFS tends to strike "suddenly and is relentless or relapsing, causing tiredness or easy fatigability in someone who has no apparent reason for feeling this way."[23]

—In 1991–92 a long-simmering dispute over the potential risks associated with silicone breast implants made headlines. As many as one million to two million American women had implants, which were employed both for cosmetic breast enlargement and for postsurgical reconstruction. Some recipients, plagued by pain, scarring, hardened tissue, silicone leakage, and other problems, deemed the product a curse. But to others implants were a psychological boost.[24]

—In late 1991 the press reported on new drug-resistant strains of tuberculosis associated with thirteen deaths in the New York prison system.[25] By the following May, the federal government had announced a plan to combat the spread of drug-resistant TB. Officials declared that TB was "out of control in the United States."[26]

—In January–February 1993 news came that hamburgers consumed at certain fast-food outlets in Washington state had been contaminated with a particular serotype of *Escherichia coli* (*E. coli* 0157:H7), a bacterium that thrives in the intestines of healthy cattle. The nearly five hundred reported cases of bloody diarrhea and hemolytic uremic syndrome in Washington were part of an eventual four-state outbreak of an illness first identified in 1982.[27]

—May 1993 brought reports of a frightening new illness in the southwestern United States, characterized by "abrupt onset of fever, myalgias, headache, and cough, followed by the rapid development of respiratory failure."[28] By June 21, eighteen persons had died from what would be formally labeled hantavirus pulmonary syndrome (HPS), acquired from rodent droppings.[29]

Emergent Public Health Hazards

Despite their many differences, these episodes share certain general characteristics that make them a distinctive challenge to policymakers, especially at the federal level. Each is an example of an *emergent public health hazard*, which is an infectious disease or product-associated danger with three general attributes: First, such a hazard victimizes relatively soon after exposure. Second, the potential exists for the hazard to spread, by one means or another, to many more victims far beyond the points of origin or discovery (unlike a plane crash or bridge collapse). Third, the hazard embodies a large measure of novelty, which facilitates uncertainty and even panic. The hazard that is new or newly recognized or suddenly ascendant as a matter of public anxiety is a

special challenge.[30] In the more persistent and better-publicized episodes, a nationwide apprehension prevails. Tangible victimization is
generally restricted, but a secondary "epidemic of fear" is always a
possibility and usually far more widespread.[31]

One important reason for the fear triggered by these hazards is that
even a single encounter with a causal agent can inflict serious harm.
A single sex act or exposure to tainted blood can transmit the HIV that
leads to AIDS.[32] One tick bite can result in Lyme disease. A single
vaccination may, if only in extremely rare instances, maim the recipient
it is intended to protect. One toxic pill can kill. By engaging in the
wrong behavior even once, a person may become a victim—a fact that
is often unknown at the outset but that sharply intensifies anxiety once
widely perceived.[33]

Most of the contentious regulatory and health issues that policymakers face, and that the public learns to dread, stem from disorders that
are a long time in the making. Neither lung cancer nor emphysema
develops from smoking a single cigarette; smoking-related ailments do
not appear within days or weeks of taking up the habit. One trip into
a coal mine does not bring on the dreaded black lung. Workers exposed
to cotton dust are not thought to face serious risk from one day on the
job. Long-term or continuing exposure is linked to the perceived harm.
Partly because of this, such threats more easily invite prolonged controversy about the size and severity of the risks in question—including
claims that they may be minimal or nonexistent. How much is too
much? How many are too many? Three long-prominent environmental
issues (acid rain, ozone layer depletion, and global warming) exemplify
this characteristic, as does the more recent debate over the potential
risk posed by electromagnetic fields.[34]

Some discrete threats inspire at least brief bouts of public fear without claiming any identifiable victims. In 1989 an environmental advocacy group, the Natural Resources Defense Council (NRDC), triggered
a national panic over apples. As a result of skillful media management,
an NRDC-sponsored report on the cancer risk that pesticides pose to
children garnered national attention. The most prominent chemical
villain was Alar, a substance used to keep apples on trees longer.
Industry revenues plummeted as shoppers and school lunch programs
refused to buy apples. Ultimately, after millions of dollars in industry
losses, and despite government assurances that apples were safe to

eat, Alar was withdrawn from the market. The scare yielded a major epidemic of fear but no identifiable victims of Alar.[35]

The emergent public health hazard is different. It claims authentic and visible victims, not invisible or hypothetical ones. The costs of inaction are thus immediate because further victimization seems imminent. Moreover, the costs of taking definitive action usually appear to be readily manageable, which is not the case for such hugely expensive international problems as acid rain, ozone layer depletion, and global warming.

These conditions have at least two important implications for policymaking. First, interminable debate over whether a genuine threat exists is far less likely. Deferral politics, both common and tempting for a wide array of environmental hazards posing largely hypothetical long-term risks (and potentially astronomical abatement costs), is largely foreclosed. Second, a special burden resides with government officials, who must focus on the new target risk relatively quickly while attending to competing needs, including forestalling far more serious risks. One of the most vexing challenges confronting policymakers is that threats of this sort yield effects that are often both serious and yet comparatively rare, perhaps the most important facet of the urgency and restraint balancing problem.[36]

Two well-established insights apply strongly to the circumstance of emergent public health hazards. The first is that newly recognized, rare, unfamiliar, or involuntarily borne risks often appear more threatening than those that are familiar or taken on willingly.[37] Diseases that generate sudden, and perhaps unpredictably recurring, epidemics have long been viewed differently from those that are endemic. One historian of public health remarked that in the early nineteenth century "the dread of yellow fever, plague, and cholera galvanized city authorities into action," while "more common endemic diseases with less spectacular lethal capacities" such as typhus, diphtheria, and tuberculosis "were met with a stolid indifference born of familiarity and a sense of helplessness."[38]

The second insight is that the visibility of victims—and their distribution in time, by area, or by various social or demographic categories—may be more significant for policymaking than their absolute numbers might suggest. In discussing the rule "Do no direct harm," economist Charles L. Schultze noted the common tendency to adjust policies that would impose high overt losses on particular firms or groups, even when the total number of persons adversely affected is comparatively small.³⁹ Political scientists have long been aware of the same dynamic, rooted largely in uneven distributions of both incentives and resources. Historians and sociologists concerned with science and disease often ground their work in "social constructionism," emphasizing the larger context of ideas and values through which people present or interpret illness. Diseases, victims, and scientific specialists may all embody particular attributes, apart from morbidity and mortality rates, that profoundly affect the way an illness is "constructed" or "framed" by society.⁴⁰ In an earlier era, well before the germ theory had revolutionized the analysis of disease, infection was commonly thought less likely to strike the virtuous, while undesirables and the lower classes were deemed especially prone to succumb.⁴¹ Even now certain classes of persons, such as children and the elderly, are seen as deserving, while homosexuals and drug abusers may, from an uncharitable perspective, get what they deserve. The strong linkage of AIDS (and other sexually transmitted diseases) to perceptions of appropriate conduct and deservedness reflects the moral claims that remain deeply relevant to health policymaking, no matter how much researchers and other professionals might crave refuge in science, technology, and moral neutrality. Cognitive psychologists report that, given a discrete choice, individuals are generally more determined to avoid a negative outcome than to pursue a positive outcome of equal magnitude.⁴² As the mass media and the popularity of health and safety in poll results suggest, Americans are extremely health-conscious—though they do not always behave accordingly. High sensitivity to risks (especially when novel or involuntarily borne) and to losses (particularly when tangible) help make emergent public health hazards, as a general category of problem, especially compelling for both policymakers and the public.

It is worth emphasizing that although emergent hazards victimize concretely in the near term, unlike many carcinogens, uncertainty and ambiguity abound. The technical and political charge to policymakers to resolve or cope with uncertainty is challenging partly because the consequences of failure are often both conspicuous and easily dramatized.

This book concludes by briefly restating key findings and reviewing the limited options available for enhancing response to such hazards. The problem of emergent hazards forces an examination of the appropriate levels of anticipatory and reactive policymaking. Is society better off trying to anticipate and prevent potential dangers or responding creatively to manifest ones? While allowing that both have a role to play, political scientist Aaron Wildavsky argued vigorously that society stresses anticipation excessively while insufficiently encouraging creative reaction (or what he called "resilience").[43] Emergent public health hazards are case studies in attempted creative reaction. While anticipation and reaction might appear easy to distinguish from one another, the two actually blend. Concrete victimization unleashes a focused reaction as well as prevention-prone sentiment and political energy. A primary significance of emergent hazards lies not in the management of the episodes themselves but in the wider and more durable reassessments and reforms they trigger. Little choice exists but to emphasize (fast) resilience against emergent public health hazards in general. Partly because the present argument concentrates on a somewhat different set of risks than Wildavsky examined, its tone is less aggressively skeptical. Wildavsky and other critics of anticipation and regulatory stringency are primarily concerned with kinds of harms that are exceedingly unlikely overall, such as nuclear power plant meltdowns. This book examines dangers that are unlikely to afflict most persons but that are not, by definition, utterly hypothetical.

The Special Problem of AIDS

AIDS occupies a prominent place in this book. The epidemic is uniquely complex and, among the problems discussed here, is the only authentic long-term national and international crisis. It has yielded an extraordinary range of political and practical difficulties, stretching across each phase of policy response. Case definitions, surveillance, epidemiologic studies, biomedical science, regulatory policy, preventive education—none of these has proved a straightforward matter for very long. No other episode considered in this book has created such uncertainty and controversy ranging across all of the key tasks under consideration. The variety of HIV-related problems is staggering: a threatened blood supply; adult versus pediatric AIDS; injection drug abuse; a synergistic relationship with tuberculosis; concerns of morality and discrimination, and so on. Each newly recognized mode of potential transmission has generated a new set of difficult policy choices. Although the possibility of patient-to-health worker transmission of HIV had been an issue for several years before 1990–91, it was only then that the public became aware of the case of David Acer, the Florida dentist who apparently transmitted the virus on the job. That revelation set off a wave of fear and debate about the possible dangers patients faced.

If AIDS is so special, why include it with other problems that are, on the whole, much less severe and forbidding? While the nature of AIDS is taken for granted today, it was not always thus. The first *New York Times* account of the epidemic, dated July 3, 1981, was headlined "Rare Cancer Seen in 41 Homosexuals" and buried deep inside the paper.[44] Only in 1982 had the first handful of transfusion-associated cases begun to surface, and by the following year the disease had become a reportable condition in every state.[45] Moreover, separate facets of response to the epidemic—field investigation, say, or regulatory issues—can be usefully discussed in comparison with other problems in the search for telling similarities and differences. Examining the HIV issue in this way helps to highlight the broad array of problems and responses that emergent public health hazards as a whole produce. A general class of hazard problem exists that is much broader than its most conspicuous and challenging example. Often, discussions of AIDS refer only briefly to lesser public health emergencies, usually to make the point that the government seemed to respond more quickly and wholeheartedly to them than to AIDS.[46] While largely true as far as they go, such unbalanced and partial accounts can also distort reality, thus poorly serving both policy debate and public understanding. For in crucial ways, lesser problems like Legionnaires' disease and toxic shock syndrome were quite different from AIDS. But bringing the tools of biomedical science to bear quickly and effectively on any infectious disease can be difficult. Similarly, problems in field inquiry, regulatory policy, education, and behavior modification are not unique to AIDS. And however unpleasant it might be to contemplate, another new infectious disease may someday supersede AIDS in significance.

The media and AIDS activists often interpret response to the disease in terms of heroes and villains, a natural result of the way journalists and policy advocates function. The rhetoric and imagery of heroism and villainy serves their respective needs. But this tendency can obscure some old lessons that AIDS teaches anew. For the student of government institutions and policymaking, those lessons are less about heroism or villainy than about other things. One is the way such forces as knowledge (or the lack of it), structures, procedures, and institutional or political incentives combine to drive activity. Another is the considerable difficulty of turning such activity into a desired outcome. Because prospects for successful policy intervention hinge so strongly on a hazard's fundamental technical and political characteristics, institutional and procedural reforms intended to cope with an existing problem, or to anticipate future ones, are blunt and problematic instruments.

Two

Institutions

T HE INVOLVEMENT of multiple institutions complicates policymaking. Federal agencies must interact with several
important external actors to cope with emergent public health hazards.
The federal bureaucracy is itself diverse and may be hard to coordinate
effectively, particularly against any large and multifaceted problem.
No federal official or office controls more than a portion of the relevant
machinery. Even the president of the United States lacks the ability,
and usually the incentive, to play any active, ongoing role in hazard
management.

Policy Actors

Four external actors play particularly significant roles in the shaping
of public policy in response to an emergent hazard: state and local
health officials, politicians, interest groups and their constituents, and
the press.

STATE AND LOCAL HEALTH OFFICIALS. State and local pub-
lic health agencies are as noteworthy for their diversity of structure,
procedure, and priorities as for their frontline position in the battle for
public health.[1] This diversity is a familiar double-edged sword,
allowing responsiveness to local interests and sensitivities while foster-
ing unsettling inequalities across jurisdictions. An Institute of Medicine
committee charged with a broad assessment of the American public
health system observed:

> In one state the committee visited, the state health department was
> a major provider of prenatal care for poor women; in other places,
> women who could not pay got no care. Some state health depart-

ments are active and well equipped, while others perform fewer functions and get by on relatively meager resources. Localities vary even more widely: in some places the local health departments are larger and more sophisticated technically than many state health departments. But in too many localities, there is no health department. Perhaps the area is visited occasionally by a "circuit-riding" public health nurse—and perhaps not.[2]

Whatever the condition of state and local systems, the federal government has little choice but to work with and through them. Federal authorities rely on state and local agencies to collect data, to assist in identifying and investigating disease outbreaks, and to deliver goods and services pursuant to national health objectives. In the areas of immunization and control of tuberculosis and sexually transmitted diseases, the federal Centers for Disease Control and Prevention provides funds to the states. In fiscal year 1992, for example, the agency awarded more than $145 million in HIV/AIDS prevention project funds to facilitate state and local efforts, while sexually transmitted disease grants totaled $77.5 million.[3]

Because an emergent health hazard is often a localized or geographically skewed problem, the administrative and political burdens for particular state and local agencies, and their leaders, may be intense. Lyme disease has been a far higher priority for New York and Connecticut health agencies than for most other states or for the nation as a whole, despite the occasional surge of national publicity. Although a local or regional disease outbreak, such as the 1993 Washington state epidemic of bloody diarrhea caused by consumption of bacteria-contaminated hamburger, may have national public policy significance in the long run, its immediate burdens fall almost entirely on the jurisdictions of tangible victimization.[4] Even the HIV epidemic has remained a relatively modest problem in many places (notably the rural West and Midwest, where infection rates remain strikingly low), while overtaxing public health resources in such locales as New York, San Francisco, Miami, Houston, and other cities. Before AIDS, subnational public health agencies, even in big cities, performed tasks that tended to strike most politicians, and most of the public, as noncontroversial and routine. As one observer commented:

> [State and local] public health executives did not serve, or at least were not perceived to be serving, a particularly unattractive or

unpopular clientele before the mid-1980s. If anything, public health executives were in the business of protecting the "public good," and their actions typically did not provoke either intense support or intense opposition. Activities such as the conduct of epidemiological surveillance, the regulation of food establishments, or even the enforcement of quality assurance in health facilities do not directly engage clients or constituencies that are highly stigmatized, nor are they activities that raise the questions of deservedness or moral hazard that are prevalent in the administration of social services or corrections agencies. . . .

Public health officials, generally medical doctors with additional public health credentials, also have benefited from the sovereignty and authority of these professions. Most issues of public health are technically and scientifically complex, and administrators with specialized expertise (or access to that expertise) in fields such as epidemiology or toxicology have enjoyed considerable hegemony over their enterprise and received substantial deference from legislators, budget officers, and the executive branch.[5]

The advent of AIDS changed this political environment, thrusting many public health executives "into the eye of the storm."[6] The HIV epidemic would prompt more aggressive efforts by the CDC to influence local disease prevention through additional—and conditional— federal funding. But many controversies (such as whether to close gay bathhouses, distribute clean needles to injecting drug users, or promote condom use) would remain local issues as much as, or more than, federal ones. Federal officials could not single-handedly determine where a balance of urgency and restraint would be struck or keep AIDS from becoming an issue far beyond public health.

POLITICIANS. Elected officials constitute the most directly important reservoir of demands, resources, rewards, and sanctions for public agencies in their respective jurisdictions. And in a federal system, politicians at one jurisdictional level may also make claims against resources, or otherwise try to shape governmental behavior, in another. Whether legislators or executives, politicians will perceive an imminent health hazard as a possible opportunity or potential threat, depending on at least a rough judgment of the chances for harvesting credit or blame. Each politician confronts a somewhat different universe of demands and needs, and embodies a distinctive set of basic competencies and stylistic attributes, from every other. Each will face much competition for his or her attention while having to nurture ongoing alliances and sources of support. Therefore the incentive and opportunity to become involved in an issue, and the nature of that involvement, can vary greatly among politicians. A legislator identified with health concerns, dependent upon health-focused constituencies, and possessing some formal claim to policy leadership (via committee or subcommittee chairmanship) will be best positioned to identify an emergent hazard as worthy of political attention, to scrutinize agency response, to offer credible assessments of official performance, and to promote favored policy reforms. Conspicuous in Congress have been such figures as Representatives Henry A. Waxman, Democrat of California, chairman of the Subcommittee on Health and the Environment of the House Committee on Energy and Commerce; John D. Dingell, Democrat of Michigan, chairman of the House Committee on Energy and Commerce and of its Subcommittee on Oversight and Investigations; Ted Weiss, Democrat of New York, chairman of a key subcommittee of the House Committee on Government Operations; and Senator Edward M. Kennedy, Democrat of Massachusetts, chairman of the Labor and Human Resources Committee. (Weiss died in 1992.)

Presidents tend to keep a low profile on emergent public health hazards. In one sense they are like the typical member of Congress, having little to gain and too much competition for their time. Exceptions occurred in 1976, when President Gerald R. Ford personally announced the swine flu program, and in 1987, when President Ronald Reagan ended years of official silence on the AIDS epidemic to deliver a speech on the eve of the third international conference on AIDS. In both cases, visible presidential involvement stemmed from a perception by the White House that the risks (political and otherwise) of inaction had become unacceptably high. Whatever his level of visibility, the president usually confines himself to statements of reassurance.

The presence of identifiable victims may either offer ammunition to the politician seeking to highlight a threat for peers and the public or create an obstacle to one with alternative priorities. During the early and mid-1980s congressional Democrats sought to pressure the Reagan administration toward greater funding for, and faster response to, both the AIDS epidemic and their health agenda more generally. For them, the availability of immediate victims offered leverage, a way to make these concerns concrete. For conservative lawmakers and the White

House, the presence of the victims was an obstacle to efforts to spotlight alternative policy interests, to control spending, and to avoid caving in to organized homosexuals.

For many politicians, however, the presence of victims will be less the means to a preestablished set of policy goals than an open opportunity to become identified with a new issue—a threat raising fear among constituents and an expectation that the government will do whatever it can to manage the problem. An emergent hazard's primary impact is strongly reflected in the pattern of concern shown by politicians. Not surprisingly, politicians with large and active gay constituencies were among the first to call for increased attention to the AIDS epidemic, and evidence of heterosexual transmission would prove crucial to galvanizing the attention and support of politicians without such constituencies. Pennsylvania politicians were understandably at the forefront during and after the deadly outbreak of Legionnaires' disease in Philadelphia in 1976. Similarly, politicians both in New York state and throughout the New England region have generally manifested the greatest awareness of and concern about Lyme disease.[7]

But politicians face powerful constraints. They want to avoid taking positions unpopular with constituents. They tend to be generalists, lacking in the technical training and knowledge necessary for deep comprehension of many problems. Their second-guessing of professionals and government agencies may be ill-informed or superficial, particularly when evaluated by experts. The separation between policy decisions and policy implementation means that members of Congress and their staffs must rely both on what they are told about agency performance and on trying to create incentives for effectiveness and truthfulness by agency officials. (It also means that legislators can generally avoid blame for implementation failures.) This separation and the prevalence of legal training among legislators combine with political incentives to give legislative oversight of the bureaucracy a strongly procedural, and sometimes prosecutorial, orientation. Procedural integrity, or the lack of it, is easy for members of Congress to comprehend and to make comprehensible to others. Concern for procedural integrity and a finely tuned sensitivity to constituent anxieties (actual or potential) are hallmark themes of legislative oversight.[8] (The two themes can lead in contradictory directions. Politicians commonly preach procedural fidelity while urging exceptions or flexibility for favored interests.) When politicians can plausibly link faulty process to concrete victimization, they generate political blame and, possibly, a full-blown scandal. Agency officials are well aware of all these things and of the need to tread carefully to preserve political support and administrative autonomy. The technical nature of emergent hazards, combined with a perception of emergency, helps protect agencies, but only imperfectly.

INTEREST GROUPS AND THEIR CONSTITUENTS. The availability of victims can either serve as fodder for existing groups and their leaders or constitute the basis for entirely new organizations. In the former instance, the incentive will be much as it is for politicians, with whom group leaders often forge alliances. Victims capture attention and inspire sympathy, thus providing visibility for groups and their preferred causes. A group anxious to advance a more general criticism will seize on a problem that group leaders can employ to reinforce a broader agenda. Groups may use emergent hazards in this way. Public Citizen, the advocacy organization founded by Ralph Nader, did this with Reye's syndrome, toxic shock syndrome, and other episodes during the 1980s.[9] For advocacy organizations reliant on generating public alarm to counteract the inherently advantaged position of business interests in routine policymaking, a new hazard (or newly frightening information about an old one) may help capture the sympathetic attention of politicians, the press, and the public. Such an issue may also have implications for the internal life of the group, allowing leaders to mobilize followers, fend off challengers, and increase the resources available for enhancement of group activity. An irony visible throughout political life is that harm to a group's constituency can augment the power of the group itself.

Victims, their friends, and relatives may also organize to affect the agendas and political environments of decisionmakers. Dalkon Shield victims and parents of children claiming harm by the diphtheria-pertussis-tetanus (DPT) vaccine, infant formula, or aspirin-associated Reye's syndrome may lobby or litigate or employ other avenues in search of redress and policy change they believe will benefit them or prevent further victimization.[10] (The same phenomenon has occurred among families whose members have been killed in terrorist bombings or declared missing-in-action in war.) Moreover, grassroots organizations are more inclined to strong emotional appeals, and sometimes even militant antiestablishment protest, than are the more traditional health lobbies. Former Federal Trade Commission chairman Michael Pertschuk observed that "the organizational culture of [traditional] voluntary associations like the [American] Cancer Society is shaped by their dependence upon the support of business leaders. Much of the staff and many of the volunteer leaders are simply not comfortable taking an aggressive, adversarial stand against any segment of the business community, nor with any form of political advocacy other than support for research funding."[11] Organized persons with breast cancer, Alzheimer's disease, and, most conspicuously, AIDS have on occasion proved less restrained.[12]

Finally, a variety of organizations representing business and professional constituencies become active in the politics of emergent hazards. Manufacturer participation arises on at least two fronts: the defense of established products and the availability of new ones. When products in general use come under attack, efforts are made to fend off adverse regulation. In recent years, business has faced demands to develop AIDS treatments and to make them available cheaply. Various health care providers (for example, physicians and hospitals) may also seek influence over policy. The Pharmaceutical Manufacturers Association (PMA) is a primary player on research and regulatory issues affecting the drug industry. The best-known lobby of professionals is the American Medical Association (AMA), a group with the reputation of being resourceful enough to eschew formal coalitions.

The political significance of interest groups lies largely in the rewards and sanctions they provide politicians (though the precise role of interest group money on the policy-relevant behavior of politicians is a matter of some dispute). While it would be misleading to think of politicians as mere empty vessels into which interest groups pour their assorted preferences, the drive for reelection is clearly important to how elected officials behave, and group evaluations can be crucial.[13] Politicians may hold relatively weak personal preferences on many issues, such as questions of administrative structure and procedure, which groups tend to perceive as vital to their interests. "To the extent this holds true [of politicians]," political scientist Terry M. Moe observed, "their positions on issues are not really their own but are induced by the position of others."[14] Groups and constituents (individuals, state governments and their agencies, business firms) also lobby agencies directly. When appealing to politicians seems too risky or otherwise unpromising, a group may have to make its position known before an agency without the oversight or casework that legislators provide. And where lobbies are divided or otherwise weak, their individual members may have strong incentives to proceed on their own.

Organized interests also go to court. The judicial role in emergent public health hazards stems from the incentives and resources of parties in judicial proceedings, the constraining influence of past decisions, and the power of judges to make law where statutes remain unclear. Aggrieved individuals and groups resort to the courts to defend claimed rights and to compel agencies to act or refrain from acting. Because judicial decisionmaking focuses so closely on rights and procedural correctness in particular cases, it is not a forum that should be expected to settle satisfactorily questions of urgency and restraint or of technical competence.[15]

THE PRESS. A key aim of politicians and interest groups is obtaining favorable media attention. While points of tension exist among them, all three institutions function in tacit alliance out of mutual self-interest.[16] Reporters need groups and politicians as sources for stories and commentary. Groups and politicians seek public outlets to shape issues and perceptions of themselves. One commentator remarked that "the press plays an influential mediating role in the policy process by selecting, packaging . . . and passing on to the public risk assessments generated and framed by scientists, the government, industry, and advocacy groups, and by reflecting back to these groups the public's response."[17]

In health and science, reporters and editors are particularly drawn to four kinds of stories, which can be labeled fire alarms, breakthroughs, controversies, and human interest.

Fire alarm stories call attention to a hazard, such as a deadly meningitis outbreak on a college campus.[18] Press accounts may also highlight new scientific findings that attach risks to activities widely believed innocuous, such as coffee consumption. The untutored layperson getting brief, incomplete, and out-of-context accounts of scientific findings can be forgiven a fair amount of confusion about what to believe or take seriously, which is particularly distressing given the importance of the media as a source of important health information.[19] A National Cancer Institute (NCI) survey found that about 60 percent of respondents relied on newspapers, magazines, and television as their main sources of information about cancer prevention, while only 15 percent or less talked to physicians about it.[20]

Scientific breakthroughs attract press coverage, which usually offers little solace to disease victims because a new treatment is too limited or comes too late to help them or because the new knowledge reported is still a long way from usable technology. Most reports of AIDS discoveries are of this last sort, offering little or no immediate benefit to most people with AIDS.

Controversy also attracts journalists. It may involve allegations of misconduct, struggles over product labeling, or arguments over appropriate regulation. The more colorful the dynamics of attack, defense, and counterattack, the greater the coverage stimulated. Journalists also try to create controversy instead of merely reflecting it, and much investigative journalism is pursued with this in mind.[21]

Finally, victims allow reporters to inject human interest into an otherwise dry or abstract subject. The HIV epidemic and other emergent hazards have produced countless tales of personal suffering and resilience.

Not all emergent hazards will be carefully or comprehensively reported. Critics of media response to AIDS in the early years of the epidemic note that the mainstream press largely ignored what then was perceived as a "gay disease."[22] Even when reporters pay attention to a problem, biases rooted in standard operating procedures and dependence on particular technologies shape the treatment that stories receive.[23] Television news is notorious for relying on good visuals and on hooking viewers quickly to avoid defection to other broadcasts. The more accessible a story's location, the more likely it will be covered. Reporters and editors also have career ambitions and political preferences. And they may be constrained by community sensitivities and by their accountability to corporate management.

Coverage has both public health costs and benefits. As media coverage raises public awareness of a health hazard, additional persons, suddenly aware that they might be or once have been victims, may report to physicians and public health authorities, possibly skewing data collection and epidemiologic analysis in important ways.[24]

Whatever emotional investment they may have in a story, responsible journalists typically strive for at least the appearance of evenhandedness. Along with getting the facts, producing balanced coverage is highly valued and usually means getting all sides of a story (though considerable bias can creep in).[25] But emergent hazards may also raise a different sort of balancing responsibility akin to the urgency versus restraint dilemma that policymakers face. For example, having encouraged public fear with accounts that a five-month-old girl's death in late 1991 may have stemmed from tainted baby food, the New York media were then obliged to report the absence of a wider pattern of food tampering and, still later, that the infant had not died of food poisoning after all.[26] Also, reporting on a two-day meeting at the CDC devoted to the tuberculosis epidemic, *New York Times* medical writer Lawrence K. Altman produced successive accounts with contrasting headlines. The first was titled "Deadly Strain of Tuberculosis Is Spreading Fast," and the second, "For Most, Risk of Contracting Tuberculosis Is Seen as Small."[27]

Policy Mandates

The diverse policy actors interact with a federal Public Health Service (PHS) once limited to "sick or disabled seamen" and funded with a monthly tax of 20 cents extracted from a seafarer's wages.[28] When a devastating cholera epidemic struck the United States in 1832, the major federal "issue" was whether President Andrew Jackson should endorse a day of "fasting and humiliation" as an effective prophylaxis.[29] In that era, subnational jurisdictions fended for themselves. Decades of scientific and technological achievement, legislative activity, and institution-building have created a vastly larger and more complex role for government in public health. But the loose PHS umbrella that encompasses key federal agencies—including the National Institutes of Health (NIH), the Food and Drug Administration, and the Centers for Disease Control and Prevention—is far less significant for managing health hazards than the historic missions and approaches of individual agencies.

NATIONAL INSTITUTES OF HEALTH. The NIH includes twenty-five major administrative units—seventeen are institutes—which form the heart of federally sponsored biomedical research.[30] The intramural research program represents a relatively small, if prestigious, presence among the NIH's total commitments, accounting for perhaps 7 to 15 percent of spending in any given year and never more than about 30 percent in any institute. Extramural programs consume the vast majority of resources, making them, in political and substantive terms, the primary raison d'être of the agency. In fiscal year 1992, for example, Congress appropriated $10 billion for the NIH, of which $7.1 billion exited the agency as grants and contracts.[31]

Overall, the NIH is decentralized, and quick reaction to new public health hazards has not been its mission. The institutes have enjoyed substantial autonomy, organized largely around particular diseases and organs. This results from a political environment in which congressional advocates and disease lobbyists have tended to concentrate on specific ailments and to prefer the greater predictability, control, and symbolic payoff inherent in specialized research units.[32]

The existing state of affairs has proven reliable for assuring strong external support among scientists, policy advocates, and members of Congress, especially because it has appeared to facilitate scientific productivity. The NIH has thrived politically by deferring to outside scientists on review committees and in research labs regarding the paths most likely to enhance scientific knowledge, not by responding to sudden emergencies.

FOOD AND DRUG ADMINISTRATION. Keeping hazardous products off the market is largely the FDA's mission. Any public health hazard that stems from a food, food additive, drug, vaccine, or medical device will likely require FDA regulatory involvement. New drugs and devices require agency approval before marketing. The FDA's regulatory authority is also broader than its power to approve or disapprove products. The agency can attach precise conditions of approval by limiting drugs to particular ailments and requiring record-keeping and reporting. The FDA also exercises considerable regulatory authority over the information that manufacturers may or must make available to consumers, a responsibility directly relevant to emergent health hazards.

The FDA thus is in a critical position regarding many hazards, rendering it vulnerable to blame from politicians, interest groups, and the press. The FDA may either approve a substance that causes direct harm to some persons or fail to approve one for which an organized or organizable constituency exists. Vitriolic criticism by AIDS activists helped push the FDA to recast procedures to speed the review of drugs for life-threatening illnesses.[33]

The agency will find evading responsibility difficult, even though circumstances hard or impossible for it to control may contribute to the problem. Uncertainty goes with the territory, given the number of products, applications for approval, clinical trials, physicians, and individual patient outcomes the FDA must monitor. Ponderous process is largely the result of having to perform a technically complex task in a high-stakes political environment (including pharmaceutical and medical device manufacturers, farmers, health professionals, and consumer advocates), often with inadequate resources.[34] This can produce drawn-out policy battles, as with the interminable fight over six artificial food colors found to cause cancer in laboratory animals.[35] The environment of regulatory politics also accounts for why the FDA to date has lacked statutory authority to order product recalls. Many business lobbies oppose such authority as excessive and unnecessary.

CENTERS FOR DISEASE CONTROL AND PREVENTION. In contrast to the FDA, recommendations and technical assistance, not regulation, is the CDC's primary business. The agency, based in Atlanta, has cultivated a core identity and constituency as a provider of practical service to state and local public health bureaucracies, though some state and local officials complain that the CDC is insufficiently sensitive to their needs. Unlike the NIH, the CDC's research activities lean more strongly toward practical application and are almost entirely intramural.[36] Whether in immunization campaigns, epidemic investigations, laboratory analysis, or training, the CDC has been a source of funds, personnel, and advice at the state and local level.[37] Originating as an agency for malaria control in war areas during the Second World War, the CDC would be transformed into an institution with national responsibility for fighting infectious disease of all sorts. The CDC is the closest thing the nation has to an institutionalized national line of defense against sudden eruptions of disease, placing responsibility for emergent public health hazards at the heart of its mandate.

While such an agency might be expected to command virtually automatic support, the CDC's position is potentially precarious. State health agencies can be protective of their autonomy, and in its early years the CDC worked diligently to entice cooperation from state officials.[38] The agency's persistent difficulty in securing a consolidated permanent headquarters reflected its political weakness. While disease and organ constituencies (including highly motivated and attentive university-based research scientists) swelled the NIH coffers in the years after World War II, the Atlanta disease detectives labored in relative poverty. And even though the CDC is now solidly established, it remains vulnerable to the political and policy dilemmas of public health. Absent a visible health crisis, its mission has often tended to generate indifference. But when a crisis strikes, the country demands predictive and diagnostic certainty as quickly as possible. Because disease is inherently complex, its cause and course hard to foresee precisely, predictive and diagnostic failure (or, at least, delay) may occur. The resulting blame can be acute. The delicate and essential balance between urgency and restraint, difficult enough to strike in any field of policy under the best of conditions, is particularly troublesome when mass fear intrudes.

SURGEON GENERAL. The surgeon general occupies an ironic position in American public health: oldest and, formally at least, weakest.[39] The post predates much of the government—its first occupant was appointed in 1871—but its powers are today largely informal and hortatory. Despite a relatively recent loss of formal authority—until a mid-1960s reorganization, the surgeon general ran the PHS—the office retains considerable visibility as a national bully pulpit for public health.[40] During the late 1960s and early 1970s the position came under sharp attack by critics as a threat to political control by the president and the secretary of health, education, and welfare (HEW).[41] The position survived, albeit weakened. During the 1980s C. Everett Koop, a pediatric surgeon, displayed considerable energy and entrepreneurial skill handling such hot issues as cigarette smoking, abortion, and AIDS. The surgeon general remains a potentially powerful force in emergent problems (such as AIDS or RS) that are not quickly resolved by the other agencies. Politicians and interest groups recognize the latent importance of the surgeon general. That is why liberals, fearful of Koop's conservative credentials as an antiabortion crusader, opposed his nomination to the post and why conservatives, anxious about Joyce-lyn Elders's support for sex education and condom distribution, responded similarly in 1993.

ASSISTANT SECRETARY FOR HEALTH. At the apex of the Public Health Service stands the assistant secretary for health, who must bear the conflicting expectations inherent in such a position. As with similar posts, the initial appointment usually stirs little controversy.[42] But once confirmed, the assistant secretary must preside over such politically charged matters as abortion, fetal tissue research, food and pharmaceutical regulation, animal experimentation, scientific misconduct, and decisionmaking for epidemics. In the early 1980s Assistant Secretary Edward Brandt was caught between a largely Democratic Congress that wanted far more research money for AIDS and the Reagan administration's desire to hold the line on spending and fend off any identification with the political agenda of organized homosexuals.[43] During the Ford administration Assistant Secretary Theodore Cooper stood at the vortex of debate over and implementation of the ill-fated swine flu vaccine program that he strongly supported and that ultimately cost him his job.[44] Like the posts of CDC and NIH director and FDA commissioner, the position is demanding enough to have been dubbed one of the "100 toughest management and policy-making jobs in Washington."[45]

Conclusion

The organizational propensity to approach any new problem in a business-as-usual manner stems mainly from an attraction to routines, procedures, and orthodoxies anchored in experience, legitimated by specific organizational environments, and supported by formal authority or informal understanding. Such forces cannot be turned around quickly. Neither the committed agency executive nor the angry activist can radically revise a large institution overnight. And expecting organizations that have long been applauded for a particular approach to routine matters instantly and dramatically to shift basic missions, decision processes, and internal reward structures is largely futile. Organizations do not easily accommodate new and unexpected problems (such as AIDS) posing complexities that lie well beyond anything in their experience. Not surprisingly, the FDA was slow to speed up drug approvals after decades of political reinforcement for keeping dangerous drugs off the market. The CDC, lacking regulatory authority and perceiving a need to nurture cooperative relationships with state and local agencies, is inclined to swim carefully in controversial waters. And if the NIH concentrates on a basic research agenda driven mostly by university-based scientists, it is because that is what the system was designed and maintained for.

Response to emergent public health hazards may be federalized, but it is not centralized. Although unburdened by deferral politics of the sort that bedevils much environmental policymaking, and despite enjoying a strong public presumption in favor of aggressive federal action, emergent hazards arise, like most issues, in an institutional context wherein multiple actors may wield crucial direct or indirect influence. (This is not to deny or to understate the genuine cooperation routinely evident among public health officials at all levels.) Health hazards range from very difficult to relatively easy. Interaction between its technical peculiarities and its political-institutional context largely determines a hazard's place on the spectrum. Bureaucratic missions and procedures, the most significant of which not only resist change but are often quite defensible, complicate the search for effective and balanced policies to deal with emergent public health hazards.

Three

Detection

THE RECOGNITION and early field investigation of novel disease outbreaks usually raise few political hurdles for the FDA and the CDC, although technical uncertainties abound. Early in the game, health authorities at all levels typically enjoy considerable deference, operating autonomy, and public confidence. These may diminish if investigation is not immediately successful (and also later, as difficulties arise in regulation, research, and public health intervention). While a hazard is newly recognized, its identified victims few and unmobilized, and politicians and the media relatively uninformed, agencies work largely unhindered. Scanty knowledge will be fodder mostly for a small corps of specialized professionals. Initial laboratory and field inquiries usually do not threaten cherished values or institutional turf, and little or no opportunity or incentive exists for agency outsiders to claim credit or cast blame. Moreover, most investigations will quickly establish an outbreak's cause, or etiology. However, if causation proves elusive, the investigation invites second-guessing and criticism, as occurred in the wake of the Pennsylvania outbreak of Legionnaires' disease in 1976. As the AIDS epidemic evolved beyond its initial stages, field inquiry stimulated controversy as it began to raise moral concerns and affect material stakes outside disease control.

Recognizing and Reporting

The most basic role that victims play in disease control is making their conditions known to health authorities by showing acute symptoms. When multiple individuals turn up over a short period bearing similar symptoms previously absent in a population, public health officials have a clear signal to be attentive.

But federal officials do not perceive public health threats automatically. Problems must usually be brought to their attention by others, and the ways this happens are both imperfect and varied. A CDC publication noted that "clusters of health events may be identified by an ongoing surveillance system, but more often they are reported by concerned citizens or groups."[1] Observant physicians are another source. Many outbreaks of infectious disease are never detected. Yet strikingly few victims are often sufficient to provoke official attention, especially when the ailment is fatal. A hair-trigger system of response has evolved that reacts to what are often tiny numbers of identified cases. Indeed, one is hard pressed to think of a field outside public health where the adverse experiences of five or ten ordinary individuals regularly and rapidly compel the attention of top agency officials.

To recognize such episodes, both the FDA and the CDC largely rely on passive surveillance, a basic tool of epidemiology and public health policy.[2] Surveillance is "the ongoing and systematic collection, analysis, and interpretation of health data in the process of describing and monitoring a health event."[3] Another tool is the epidemiologic study, which aims, through various research designs, to identify and confirm statistical associations between population characteristics or exposures and the occurrence of specific diseases.[4]

Although the Food, Drug, and Cosmetic Act requires extensive pre-market testing, side-effects may elude investigators until after a drug or device is licensed. A postlicensing system is therefore desirable to detect and evaluate adverse reactions. This system combines voluntary and mandatory reporting. The FDA's spontaneous reporting system attempts to capture, on a continuing basis, product-related adverse experience reports from physicians and other health care providers. That part of the system is voluntary, but once drug and device manufacturers detect adverse reactions, from whatever source, they are required to report them.[5] In a June 1993 speech announcing the MEDWATCH program intended to improve adverse reaction reporting, FDA Commissioner David A. Kessler highlighted the agency's unavoidable reliance on small numbers of cases to signal larger problems:

The medical writer Berton Roueché has made a career out of documenting in the most wonderful way how medical mysteries have been unravelled because a single attentive, curious practitioner recognized a clue.

Individual practitioners can signal that something is afoot. We depend on them not only to treat the patient but to recognize that the patient may also be a messenger—carrying the message that what is happening in this case or this cluster of cases may have implications for the health of many others.[6]

The CDC also relies on both voluntary and mandatory reporting. Like product surveillance (and the CDC itself), a program of systematic national reporting for a wide variety of diseases was a postwar development.[7] According to a former CDC director, no systematic and active national surveillance for any disease existed in the United States until 1950.[8] By 1990 forty-nine diseases were considered nationally reportable to the CDC's National Notifiable Diseases Surveillance System, thus creating two stages of routine mandatory reporting: physician to state health department, state health department to the CDC. The second link in the chain is far stronger than the first, partly because of technical advances and partly because individual noncompliance is avoided. The National Electronic Telecommunications System for Surveillance (NETSS) allows for reliable computer-assisted transmission of surveillance data between the states and the CDC.[9] No comparable system links health providers to their respective state health agencies, and many private physicians are only minimally familiar either with their public health agencies or with population-based preventive approaches.

The FDA and the CDC differ regarding the political implications of surveillance for newly recognized hazards. Because the CDC does not regulate products, the agency usually cannot be blamed for having helped to create the problem to which its surveillance and intervention mechanisms respond. That is not the case for the FDA, however. As a regulatory body charged with premarketing approval, the FDA collects adverse reaction reports that agency critics can then offer as evidence that the drug or device in question should never have been approved in the first place. Underreporting for drug and device adverse experiences has proved somewhat more contentious and unsettling than for infectious diseases. This reflects the political and practical ease of holding individual manufacturers accountable for specific products, and the need to do so for regulatory purposes, compared with the futility of generating blame against physicians and their patients. Even when legally required, disease reporting by individuals is "almost never enforced."[10] Meanwhile, the General Accounting Office, an investigative and evaluative arm of Congress, has repeatedly assailed weaknesses in FDA product monitoring.[11]

A crucial, though often unappreciated, distinction also exists between deeming a condition reportable and ensuring an adequate program of surveillance. As the state epidemiologist of Oklahoma observed, "Officially designating a disease or condition as reportable is a one-time activity that simply provides a framework for surveillance. The actual surveillance for that disease or condition is an ongoing, dynamic activity that requires frequent, sustained interaction with reporting sources. A surveillance system for any disease requires nurturing, in the form of feedback and follow-up of reported cases. Although most diseases or conditions for which there is ongoing surveillance are also officially reportable, the latter is not necessary for the former to take place."[12] Novel disease outbreaks can prompt the rapid creation of ad hoc surveillance, while an official designation of reportability may be months or years away.

The overall character of state-federal relations in public health helps to moderate potential conflict over surveillance but at the cost of uneven coverage and practice. States may implement surveillance according to their own priorities, creating variation in both coverage and technique that may constrain knowledge at the national level. For example, as of mid-1992 only eighteen of the fifty states required reporting of elevated blood lead levels in adults.[13] Although the CDC initiated Lyme disease surveillance in 1982, only in 1991 did all states begin using the same case definition.[14] States require health providers to report many diseases, and "reports of some 160 diseases are now required by at least one state."[15] But, again, considerable variability exists in state organization and practice. "In some states," wrote Stephen B. Thacker and Ruth L. Berkelman of the CDC, "authority [to require disease reporting] is enumerated in statutory provisions; in others the authority . . . has been given to state boards of health; still other states require reports under both statutes and health department regulations. State reporting requirements also vary among conditions and diseases to be reported, time frames for reporting, agencies receiving reports, persons required to report, conditions under which reports are required, and penalties for not reporting."[16]

One indicator of the frank sharing of power among levels of government is the role that state epidemiologists play in determining which diseases must be reported by physicians and health care institutions as part of the national notifiable disease reporting system. Contrary to what most people would probably suspect, the CDC does not unilaterally declare a disease notifiable. Instead, the Council of State and Territorial Epidemiologists, affiliated with the Association of State and Territorial Health Officials, formally controls the list of such diseases albeit with considerable informal CDC collaboration.

Because of postmarketing surveillance through physicians and manufacturers, the occasional patient who develops a novel side-effect soon after commencing a prescribed therapy is more likely to be detected and reported than is the isolated case of communicable disease. But cases of communicable disease from which patients recover quickly and without medical intervention (for example, influenza or mild gastrointestinal illness) are particularly likely to elude reporting, and relatively low reporting rates are common for the recognized infectious diseases.[17] Some physicians are either unaware of the requirement to report particular diseases or disinclined to comply given the effort involved. Almost certainly this means that some outbreaks, including novel hazards, will be discovered late, or perhaps not at all. Outbreaks most likely to be reported are those "involving serious disease, disease associated with a short incubation period or a characteristic clinical syndrome . . . or disease affecting large numbers of people."[18] Much disease is doubtless misdiagnosed. (Ironically, one reason this may happen—though how often no one knows—is when physicians are influenced too strongly by official case definitions in making their diagnoses.)[19] Underreporting is also likely if a disease is, like AIDS, socially stigmatizing. A physician might be uncomfortable making an honest report if doing so could imply a homosexual or bisexual history for a patient.[20] Low reporting rates also derive from such factors as asymptomatic infection, ill-equipped diagnostic facilities, and laboratory error.[21]

Yet until recently (see chapter 8), public health officials and experts have professed little real alarm about the underreporting of infectious disease.[22] A senior official in the CDC's Epidemiology Program Office remarked in an interview that surveillance for *Salmonellosis*, a common and occasionally fatal food-borne ailment, probably yields only one reported case for every twenty actual cases. But, he and others argued, consistently scant reporting still allows for monitoring and analysis of disease trends.[23] Because many infectious diseases, such as chicken pox or the common cold, are relatively benign, whether they are reported or not is of little consequence. For any new or newly recognized hazard, and particularly if the risk of a serious outcome is significant, more desirable is a reporting system that can better gauge the absolute size of the threat and help locate not only potential sources of the problem but also the largest possible number of victims requiring prompt intervention. The same would be true of, say, typhoid fever or botulism poisoning. Ordinarily rarely encountered in the United States, they could result in considerable disease and death in the absence of prompt recognition and intervention. For outbreaks of this sort, remarked the CDC official, "it's a lot more important to find every single case." The fullest possible case reporting is also vital when policymakers contemplate complete eradication of an infectious disease; the successful effort to eliminate smallpox depended significantly on meticulous reporting.[24]

If underreporting is a perennial problem in discerning and analyzing epidemics, the opposite and less obvious problem, overreporting, can also bedevil analysis. The diagnostic challenge of diverse or subtle symptoms may be enhanced when a hazard receives a burst of publicity. Media attention, however useful for generating interest in a condition and thus uncovering additional new cases, may increase the likelihood of false positive reports. Physicians and patients, sensitized to an emerging problem by press accounts, may unwittingly misdiagnose symptoms. Patients may also be unable to recall, or may recall incorrectly, the precise brand, dosage, or timing of a particular product they may have used.

Some analysts argue that this poses a major pitfall for the case-control studies often employed for rare ailments. Comparisons are made between a group of persons who have a disease (the cases) and a comparable group that does not (the controls) in the search for associations between illness and other attributes.[25] Some commentators argued, for example, that the epidemiologic evidence of association between toxic shock syndrome and tampon use may have been undermined by biases in both diagnosis and reporting related to the publicity surrounding the disease.[26] Similar arguments have been raised regarding both Reye's syndrome and Lyme disease.[27] In mid-1992 an FDA advisory committee recommended the retention on the market of the world's most popular prescription sleeping pill, Halcion, partly because of a suspicious association between publicity about alleged side-effects and increased case reports.[28] In the six months after *Newsweek* magazine ran a critical cover story on the drug, adverse reaction reports increased fivefold. Such data, combined with other uncertainties surrounding the validity of adverse reaction reports, inclined the committee to keep the drug available.[29] Does an increase in case reports indicate (1) a spreading problem, (2) a change in case definition, (3) an increased propensity or ability to report, or (4) some combination of these? It is often hard to know. Unfortunately, this kind of contextual detail is usually missing from press accounts trumpeting raw disease statistics.

Perhaps the most fundamental barrier to managing a novel disease outbreak is that a requirement or request for reports of specific ailments cannot be made until they are known to exist. Particularly for communicable diseases (but to some extent for product-associated problems as well) outbreak discovery depends heavily on fortuitously clustered cases of acute illness. Sometimes, as in the case of chronic fatigue syndrome, the sentinel bureaucracies may be slow to recognize and take seriously even a clustered problem. And if the appropriate public health institutions do pay attention to a problem, there is no guarantee that the resulting response will be a correct or effective one. But without clustering by location and time, authorities may be hampered in recognizing an emerging problem. That was a key constraint in the case of the mysterious non-HIV AIDS-like syndrome resulting in a small number of identified cases that surfaced to enormous media attention at the eighth international AIDS conference in Amsterdam in the summer of 1992. Later officially dubbed idiopathic CD4+ T-lymphocytopenia, this syndrome drew abundant press coverage and triggered consternation among health officials.[30] It also led to complaints that the CDC had not moved quickly enough with a vigorous investigation, a lag born at least partly of the dispersed, unclustered character of victimization.[31]

But even clustering cannot easily overcome efforts to deemphasize or deliberately hide information. Such behavior helped the deadly Dalkon Shield, an intrauterine device, to remain on the market long after users began having pelvic inflammatory disease and septic abortions. The shield's manufacturer, A. H. Robins, repeatedly ignored or downplayed reports of adverse reactions, impeding the regulatory apparatus.[32] In another instance, the FDA was slow to receive complete information about the dangers of the Bjork-Shiley Convexo-Concave heart valve, which was prone to cracking after implantation. The Shiley company, a division of Pfizer, withheld information about both the defect and deceptive manufacturing practices.[33]

For at least three reasons, the number of recognized cases need not be large to attract official notice and concern. First, unlike the average person, the epidemiologist tends to think of an epidemic as any distinctive health problem occurring at a rate greater than normal. Hence, as a CDC director of field services once observed, "one case of smallpox would be an epidemic."[34] Second, as Commissioner Kessler's remarks suggest, scientists and physicians are acutely aware that a problem found at one location can, and probably will, arise elsewhere, especially if an infectious disease or widely distributed product is the suspected hazard.[35] Third, the public health system in the United States consists of numerous and interlocking local, state, and national government bureaucracies created and maintained largely to be sensitive to the appearance of anything unusual (although they deal mostly with events that are decidedly ordinary). State and local public health agencies and the CDC constitute a vast (though imperfect and often underfunded) network of persons trained, assigned, and rewarded for conscientious monitoring and assessment of the evolving picture of disease. Everyone is aware that failure to respond in a timely fashion to a new problem, or to the new manifestation of an old one, could be costly in a variety of ways (including the blame that perceived failure generates). All of this tends to place a certain institutional weight behind a report, from one point on the network to another, of anything new, however scarce the number of known cases.

As the seven examples briefly recounted below demonstrate, emergent health hazards have regularly commenced with a few clustered cases of something unusual. The role of chance is considerable. An ailment could well exist for years, even decades, before anyone takes particular notice. (Most infectious diseases commonly perceived as new are actually only newly encountered by particular populations.)[36] A disease might recur in occasional outbreaks (as did Legionnaires' disease) that vanish before anyone can determine a cause.[37]

ACQUIRED IMMUNODEFICIENCY SYNDROME. AIDS has been around for decades. In 1987 doctors concluded on the basis of preserved blood and tissue samples that a sixteen-year-old St. Louis boy had succumbed to the disease in 1969.[38] A twenty-five-year-old sailor had inexplicably died in 1959, but only in 1990 was AIDS determined to have been the reason.[39] By the end of 1980 some fifty-five young men in the United States had been diagnosed with infections that, only later, would be identifiable as AIDS-related.[40]

But it was not until early 1981 that Dr. Michael Gottlieb, a young immunologist at the University of California at Los Angeles, had seen his second recent case of *Pneumocystis carinii* pneumonia, a rare protozoal ailment, combined with depleted T-lymphocytes, blood cells crucial to the body's system of immune response. And the second case, like the first, had occurred in a homosexual man.[41] Soon there would be five, with cytomegalovirus as well. Such observations, occurring suddenly in members of a defined population in one state, aroused the suspicions of Gottlieb and his friend Wayne Shandera, a physician detailed to the Los Angeles area by the CDC's Epidemic Intelligence Service (EIS). Moreover, only severely compromised immune systems could succumb to such ailments. This came at about the same time as reports of multiple cases of a rare cancer, Kaposi's sarcoma (KS), ordinarily seen only in elderly men. But these victims were young.[42]

These observations led to two articles in the CDC's *Morbidity and Mortality Weekly Report* (*MMWR*) in June and July of 1981 detailing, respectively, five cases of *Pneumocystis carinii* pneumonia in California and twenty-six cases of Kaposi's sarcoma—twenty in New York and the rest in California. Commentators on the AIDS epidemic would later remark on the deliberately restrained nature of these accounts (especially the first, which made no mention of the homosexual connection in its title) as an effort to avoid sensationalizing a new "gay disease," though even the June report carried an editorial note speculating on "an association between some aspect of a homosexual lifestyle or disease acquired through sexual contact and *Pneumocystis* in this population."[43] The prevalence of sexually transmitted disease (including hepatitis B) among gay men was part of the preexisting context encouraging this early linkage between the new disease and sexual preference.[44] CDC staffers apparently neither wanted to upset the homosexual community nor to encourage antigay prejudice. In hindsight, one cost of such moderation would be a failure effectively to flag AIDS as important, causing the national media (and, initially, much of the gay community) to pay little attention to the story.[45] Even at this early stage of the AIDS epidemic, political sensitivity and the delicate balance between urgency and restraint were evident.

TOXIC SHOCK SYNDROME. Toxic shock syndrome was identified and described a full year before anyone much cared about it and
had undoubtedly been present in the human population long before
that.[46] In November 1978 James Todd at the University of Colorado
School of Medicine published an article in the journal *Lancet* describing
seven cases of a new illness, in young persons ranging in age from
eight to seventeen, which he labeled toxic shock syndrome. Symptoms
included fever, low blood pressure, vomiting, a severe rash, and "fine
desquamation" or peeling of the skin on the hands and feet. Five of
the victims recovered fully; there was one case of gangrene and one
death. Todd determined that staphylococcus bacteria probably had
generated a toxin that triggered the symptoms. As one commentator
would later note, "a few isolated case reports, stretching back to 1927,
had described vaguely similar illnesses, but there had never been a
cluster with such distinct and striking symptoms."[47]

Nevertheless, little attention was paid to TSS until late 1979 and
early 1980. The real saga of TSS, which would stimulate intense press
coverage and a long regulatory battle during the 1980s, began in Wisconsin during the waning months of 1979 when a doctor encountered
three patients harboring the same symptoms that Todd had described.
As one observer would later put it, "Three cases in one week for a
very rare new syndrome seemed so unusual that [the physician] called
in the state health department epidemiologist to investigate."[48] And
unlike the children and teenagers Todd had seen—state officials then
had thought of TSS as a childhood ailment—these and later cases
included adult women, most of whom had become ill during their
menstrual periods. The Minnesota and Wisconsin state health agencies
began reporting cases to the CDC and established formal epidemiological surveillance. This, combined with considerable publicity, began to
yield still more cases, and a hunt for the cause and extent of the TSS
epidemic was on.

SWINE FLU. In January 1976 an outbreak of respiratory disease
occurred among army recruits at Fort Dix, New Jersey. Hundreds were
affected.[49] The state public health laboratories analyzed the throat wash-
ings of several recruits, identifying some as the virulent type A influenza. When the state labs were unable to specify further the precise
character of some virus samples, they were sent to the CDC. (Meanwhile, one recruit, Private David Lewis, prematurely left his sickbed,

collapsed, and died after participating in a five-mile night march.) The CDC turned up swine influenza among the samples, ominous news given the virulence of that particular subtype, associated with the so-called Spanish influenza pandemic that killed more than 20 million persons throughout the world in 1918—19. Even though any comparison with the earlier catastrophic pandemic was deliberately played down by most government officials, the news media emphasized it. In the end, Private Lewis and a dozen other persons in the United States would be the only confirmed human cases of swine flu, some of these traceable to contact with pigs.[50] Yet the small number of cases quickly prompted a strong recommendation by CDC Director David J. Sencer (supported by a largely deferential advisory committee on immunization practices) for a $135 million emergency immunization program to combat an anticipated epidemic. President Ford not only accepted the recommendation but personally announced the new program (embracing the comparison with the prior pandemic) less than two weeks after Sencer's recommendation.

LYME DISEASE. Like AIDS and TSS, Lyme disease had been around for a considerable time before its rise to prominence. Its characteristic rash (erythema chronicum migrans) and an array of secondary symptoms had become an inconspicuous part of the European medical literature in the several decades before the 1970s, when two Connecticut women separately began prodding the public health establishment about persistent problems in their own families. One of the women, Judith Mensch living in Old Lyme, would not accept the diagnosis of juvenile rheumatoid arthritis that doctors had offered to explain the crippling inflammation that beset her daughter, partly because three other children living nearby had been given the same diagnosis. Meanwhile, Polly Murray's family living in nearby Lyme suffered similar troubles.

In the fall of 1975 the women finally got both sympathy and help from Allen Steere, a physician doing postgraduate research at the Yale School of Medicine, and David Snydman, then acting epidemiologist at the Connecticut Department of Health Services. The two men were not only acquainted but also had professional ties to the CDC's EIS. Steere began to treat patients with the mysterious ailment and to collect data. The concentration of cases, and their symptoms, led him to conclude that it was not any previously identified form of arthritis. Moreover, the pattern seemed to suggest an insect-borne disease. The concentration was crucial to Steere's pursuit of the disease and to his belief that it was something out of the ordinary. "It really was marked by clusterings," he would say later. "On some streets it was one house after another. I can't tell you how different that is from [juvenile rheumatoid arthritis]. I had been given a list of names to telephone. Once I dialed the wrong number and got a home where the kid had arthritis."[51] Ecological and demographic changes in the area may have promoted this clustering, thus setting the stage for recognition of a new disease. According to one observer, "[T]he near simultaneous presentation of cases from the same geographical area presenting to Yale rheumatologists and Groton dermatologists in 1975 suggests that a threshold of biological and social circumstances had been reached, allowing recognition of a new biological process, although just what was new was open to negotiation."[52]

INFANT FORMULA. In the summer of 1979 Dr. Shane Roy, a pediatric nephrologist in Memphis, Tennessee, saw three infants suffering from hypochloremic metabolic alkalosis, a condition leading to appetite loss and general failure to thrive, triggered by insufficient levels of chloride and potassium in the blood.[53] Roy "considered the occurrence of three such cases within a period of one month in one geographic area to be highly unusual."[54] He determined that each of the victims had been nourished solely on Neo-Mull-Soy, a soy-based formula produced by Syntex Laboratories. Roy called Syntex, which said it had no other reports of a problem. But when the local health department reported the hospital admissions of Roy's patients to the CDC, the federal agency surveyed pediatric nephrologists. That survey found thirty-one cases of metabolic alkalosis, twenty-six of them in children sustained on Neo-Mull-Soy.

L-TRYPTOPHAN. In the autumn of 1989 three New Mexico women, two from Santa Fe and one from Los Alamos, were found to have "extremely high counts of a white blood cell called an eosinophil. The syndrome is known as eosinophilia."[55] Physicians treating the women contacted a recognized authority on eosinophilia, Dr. Gerald J. Gleich of the Mayo Clinic in Rochester, Minnesota. All three women had been taking the diet supplement L-tryptophan. Almost immediately, suspicion arose that L-tryptophan might be implicated. As Gleich noted at the time, "Lightning can strike, but it doesn't strike twice. . . . It could be a red herring, but a red herring in three people? I'm not willing to buy that. I'm trained to look for unexpected associations. Once is chance, twice is kind of interesting, but three and I say full speed ahead [for an investigation]."[56]

CHRONIC FATIGUE SYNDROME. Chronic fatigue syndrome has also probably been around for many years.[57] Two young physicians in the resort community of Incline Village, Nevada, discerned among local high school teachers what appeared to be a persistent flu. But, as one source later recounted, "within a few months, nearly 200 of the town's 20,000 residents had developed the same symptoms, and no one seemed to get better. Most of the sufferers were mass-producing antibodies to Epstein-Barr, the herpes virus that causes infectious mono-nucleosis. But mononucleosis is rare in adults and *epidemics* of adult mono are unheard of."[58] In this instance, it took considerable prodding to get the CDC to pay attention, but in September 1985 the agency sent two investigators, who decided that, while they could not pinpoint the precise problem, Epstein-Barr was very possibly a red herring. At about the same time, an apparent outbreak of a similar condition occurred in the vicinity of Lyndonville, New York. Both the state health department and the CDC proved reluctant to get involved, and a local physician, Dr. David Bell, and his wife, an infectious disease specialist, began to conduct a study (ultimately inconclusive) of their own. By late 1987 additional outbreaks had captured the attention of researchers around the country leading to a national conference on the illness.

Mobilizing

Important new clusters of illness are rare, which perhaps is one reason that the CDC was initially reluctant to pursue its first leads on chronic fatigue syndrome. The vast majority of infectious diseases that physicians and ordinary citizens will encounter (for example, measles, *Salmonellosis*, syphilis, gonorrhea, hepatitis) are common and familiar problems. So are many toxic substances. The existence and overall character of a problem are often relatively well understood, with both official concern and routines of response firmly established, at least in principle. This would apply as well to the yearly handful of victims of such formerly common diseases as diphtheria, cholera, or plague, made rare in the United States through immunization or improved sanitation.[59]

Occasionally, a previously unknown condition may erupt or progress largely unseen by health authorities and the public until its sudden discovery. When such a problem affects few or widely dispersed persons, a measure of sentinel advocacy (on the part of scientists, physicians, government officials, or perhaps victims themselves) may be necessary to build awareness and promote action.

The precise origins and character of sentinel advocacy will be as diverse as the diseases that trigger it. CDC Director Sencer's toughly worded memo arguing for an immediate and costly national effort to impede swine influenza was critical to capturing the attention of his superiors in the Department of Health, Education, and Welfare and in the White House. Also vital, though less sophisticated or well-positioned, was the dogged persistence of the early victims and investigators of Lyme disease in Connecticut. And Lyme disease victims' sense of frustration and fear gave them a different perspective from that leading a university-based immunologist to call attention to a few aberrant cases of *Pneumocystis carinii* pneumonia.

Reliance on sentinel advocacy, however judicious or grounded in professional judgment, raises a dilemma for policy response. Getting the attention of institutions, their members, and the public for a new problem means creating concern, perhaps alarm or outrage. But response demands considerable caution and restraint in both interventions and public pronouncements. This is especially true in the case of a newly recognized hazard that appears both serious and either rare or only occasionally life-threatening.

The response dilemma confronted CDC decisionmakers and their political superiors regarding swine flu. Does a cluster of influenza cases indicate a larger epidemic to follow? And if it does, how large will the epidemic be, and how virulent the organism responsible? In any case, what should be the policy response? The government could not have reliably predicted that swine flu would not materialize as a national epidemic, nor anticipated an epidemic of serious side-effects associated with the vaccine. The FDA felt compelled to evaluate even the now-infamous and far more clearly dangerous Dalkon Shield in light of its risks and its benefits, and in comparison with the risk-benefit profile of alternative contraceptives.

The easy part, however, is assigning personnel to a problem, commencing an investigation, and instituting what CDC officials have called "a quickly implemented ad hoc reporting system" that may evolve into a more "formal, national network involving extensive collaboration between the CDC and state and territorial health departments."[60] Once health officials had grasped the existence of toxic shock syndrome among women and AIDS among homosexual men, the CDC's most straightforward steps were the assignment of field staff to collect data and the creation of agency task forces responsible for investigative coordination and analysis. The CDC can quickly send members of its renowned Epidemic Intelligence Service and reassign other agency personnel to commence, or assist in, an investigation.[61] Besides the dispatch of EIS staff from headquarters in Atlanta for epidemiologic field investigations—the agency participated in some twenty-nine hundred such investigations, at the request of state, local, and international authorities between 1946 and 1987—the CDC also offers help in other forms, including "telephone consultations, on-site technical consultations or hazard evaluations, the analysis of data sent to CDC from state health agencies, and the assignment of CDC staff to state, local, or international health agencies."[62]

Mere hours may elapse before a federal presence is at work at the site of a problem. The CDC sent three EIS officers to Pennsylvania on August 2, 1976, the very day the agency got word of what would be called Legionnaires' disease. They joined two additional CDC staff, already in place, to initiate an investigation.[63] Such action has an obvious policy rationale. Outbreaks of serious disease are often elusive and fast-developing, and it makes sense, in the interest of effective investigation and disease containment, to obtain as much potentially useful data as possible quickly. Investigators will probe the memories of victims and collect blood and other fluid specimens along with environmental samples. The hazard at issue will likely turn out to be rare, or rarely identified, instead of something new—for example, the viral pneumonia psittacosis, occasionally transmitted to humans by birds.[64] And the chance of death or serious long-term consequences is often slight. But prompt response is in order nonetheless.

Promptness also has a political implication (though officials might deny or downplay it as a motivation). Concrete and visible action cultivates the good will of the politicians and of the state and local health agencies to which the CDC looks for cooperation and support.

The CDC would find its task more difficult were it to arouse the ire of those agencies, the persons who run them, and the politicians and clienteles associated with them. Placing skilled personnel in position fast at the request of states when they particularly need help makes for essential good relations (and a favorable public image) as well as good public health. Quick response is also an effective way to deflect potential blame, making it impossible for inquiring reporters and politicians to ask a potentially damning question: "Why was the CDC not there?"

In responding, however, the CDC must try to avoid either usurping a state's health jurisdiction or sowing confusion between state and local authorities. Veterans of the agency's Epidemiology Program Office noted that "under special circumstances, such as interstate or multistate outbreaks" the CDC may initiate investigations. More regularly, however, "requests for epidemiologic field assistance are made by the State Epidemiologists on behalf of the State public health agency," even though the request may have originated at the local level.[65] Given the wide variation in institutional arrangements between state and local public health agencies, and the potential for inadvertently provoking confusion and resentment of encroaching "feds," such a convention is understandable. And because national surveillance particularly depends on state and local governments and a network of hospitals, clinics, and individual physicians for cooperation, it must be sensitive to possible sources of resistance if it is to work effectively. Reporting requirements that are perceived as excessively burdensome or invasive invite noncompliance.[66]

Public health officials will more readily recognize and mobilize against a new problem when it arises in conjunction with one already on their agendas. In 1976 existing concerns about possible swine flu outbreaks helped energize response to the Pennsylvania outbreak of Legionnaires' disease. Later that year, adverse reactions to the influenza vaccine quickly became a high priority because the vaccine program itself was. More recently, any problem that emerges in connection with the HIV epidemic (for example, drug-resistant tuberculosis, the so-called non-HIV AIDS of 1992, or a new strain of HIV itself) will reap enhanced visibility as a result.[67] The overall resurgence of TB claimed attention partly because it was so apparent in persons with HIV disease and partly because it was highly concentrated where it was most likely to be noticed. One of the largest TB surges, including a highly publicized occurrence of drug-resistant TB bacteria among the prison population, occurred in the AIDS-aware media center of New York City, which saw a 45 percent increase in cases between 1980 and 1987.[68]

Distinguishing between governmental and media mobilization is important. To say that the press and the general public are largely unconcerned with a problem or uninformed about it does not imply a lack of governmental attention. While most of the public heard little or nothing of AIDS during the early 1980s, the CDC and state health agencies were continually active in tracking and describing the disease throughout that period.

Extremes of variation in media mobilization merit explanation. Why did the Legionnaires' disease outbreak of 1976 inspire so much media attention and public interest, leading the CDC to hold three formal press briefings in one week and set up three separate offices to handle different categories of telephone inquiries?[69] Years later, angry activists and commentators, critical of the federal health establishment's response to AIDS, would cite the Philadelphia epidemic (along with toxic shock syndrome, polio, and other diseases) as evidence of a double standard: the deaths of children or legionnaires are front-page news and a public health call to arms, while gay people die amidst indifference.[70]

There is more than a grain of truth in that recounting, for disease is socially constructed. In retrospect, a deadly new sexually transmitted disease such as AIDS, perceived as affecting mainly a pariah group defined by its sexuality, could never be considered solely in terms of public health or abstract indicators of mortality and morbidity. Legionnaires' disease bore no such limitation or stigma. Suddenly, albeit briefly, it seemed that anyone might be at risk from whatever was killing Pennsylvania legionnaires.

However, the national press pounced firmly on the story, quickly forcing the CDC into administrative overdrive to handle the inquiries, for many other reasons.[71] The story was concentrated around the single, easily accessible media center of Philadelphia. The disease's elusive etiology made for an exciting mystery partly because it produced a cluster of cases (and some twenty-nine unexplained deaths) right away, not spread out over months or years. This meant, among other things, that television always had something visual to capture immediately—the repeated rituals of burial and mourning. The outbreak also hit a press corps and public that had been primed by the president only a few months earlier to expect a possibly deadly influenza outbreak imminently. In the first two days after the CDC got word of the epidemic, the agency could not discount the possibility that swine flu might have hit (and before a protective vaccine could be distributed). Only thereafter could the CDC be reasonably certain that swine flu was not killing legionnaires. Perhaps most significant, unlike other disease outbreaks, the media received word of it via an organized press announcement by an American Legion official even before the state's top public health official had been informed.[72] Indeed, so virulent and far advanced was the outbreak that, by the time the CDC had its investigation under way, most of those who were to die had already succumbed.[73] Taken together, such conditions would have created an intriguing medical mystery of some duration for logistical reasons alone; public health authorities would need time (a few days at least) to get an investigation organized and implemented and to obtain the verified results of laboratory analysis. Meanwhile, press coverage of the story would stir public anxiety.

As for swine flu in comparison with AIDS, a simple but easily neglected fact deserves emphasis. At the time of the Fort Dix outbreak, swine influenza already had an established legitimacy as a recognized disease. That, after all, is precisely why the CDC lab could quickly identify it. Although some believed the CDC director's reaction excessive, it is also one reason why his memorandum proved so compelling. Whatever uncertainty existed, Sencer did not have to sail against technical uncertainty or a strong professional tide to propose that the particular strain of the influenza virus was active or that it could cause potentially serious disease. (Though there were doubts among his advisers about the wisdom of a national immunization campaign.) HIV was unknown until at least 1983, two years or more after the first cases of AIDS were identified. Some people suspected reasonably quickly that the mysterious syndrome was infectious and sexually transmitted, but not surprisingly, that view, and the policy implications flowing from it, took time to sink in both among public health officials and within a gay community that had a strong cultural (and, in some cases, financial) stake in denial.[74]

The social characteristics of early clusters of disease victims affect not only the avenues of analysis undertaken by disease investigators but also the perceptions of the press and the public. For the public, which necessarily learned about AIDS through press coverage, the problem was first a gay disease, later also one of Haitians, drug users, and hemophiliacs. This partly explains the initial failure of the press to catch on to what would ultimately become the predominant health story of the 1980s.[75] Little was known about the ailment at first, and journalists on the science beat were inclined to take their lead from the CDC's *MMWR*, a widely disseminated compendium of surveillance data, epidemiologic investigations, and public health recommendations. Given the time necessary to implement surveillance, sift through data, ferret out their implications, and report findings, the *MMWR* said nothing about the problem between August 1981 and May 1982—a nine-month gap in reporting reflected in a lack of media attention. Moreover, the pattern of victimization would leave many reporters and editors initially ignorant of AIDS, uncomfortable with it, unacquainted with anyone who had it, or anticipating little interest (or similar discomfort) among readers and viewers.

Toxic shock syndrome and the Dalkon Shield episode became women's issues, even though the first recognized cases of TSS had occurred in children of both sexes. The infant formula scares, DPT, and E-Ferol provoked particular sympathy (and the prompt interest of congressional investigators) partly because the victims were children. Unlike an epidemic tied to the intimate behavior of adult homosexuals, pediatric problems are immediately an attractive target for official concern. The sixteen hundred or so AIDS cases reported among U.S. children under the age of five by the end of the 1980s had acquired symbolic and political significance far beyond their numbers. The initial 1982 report of possible infant AIDS immediately helped to draw more national press coverage to the disease.[76]

Sources of Controversy

A review of emergent public health hazards suggests that field investigation generally resists controversy, especially in its early stages. Sometimes, however, the methods and results of investigation may resonate beyond the realm of disease control. In such an environment, significant conflict over values and expectations may develop.

CONTROVERSY OVER METHODS. Having recognized a novel health problem, investigators must first decide what symptoms constitute a case of the condition in question. Establishing a case definition can be intellectually tricky and sometimes politically sensitive, but it is vital to effective public health intervention. Surveillance and epidemiologic studies are impossible to perform unless one knows both what (or whom) to count and discount. An outbreak of a long-familiar disease may present a fairly easy target in this respect. Distinctive symptoms and familiar microbes facilitate the task. The most striking "symptom" of all, sudden and painful death in previously healthy persons, enormously simplified the task of investigators probing the Tylenol poisonings of 1982. But often, symptoms are more subtle, variable among cases, and perhaps easily misdiagnosed, as with Lyme disease or Reye's syndrome, an ailment associated with a "diverse clinical spectrum . . . and lack of specificity of . . . signs and symptoms," making it prone to being confused with other diseases.[77] The more elusive or variegated the symptoms of a disease or syndrome, the tougher the job can be of constructing the sort of carefully delimited case definition disease investigators prefer.

If the political environment includes the right kinds of interested parties, case definitions may provoke interest beyond disease control professionals. When *Pneumocystis carinii* pneumonia and Kaposi's sarcoma began appearing in gay men, the CDC Task Force on Kaposi's Sarcoma and Opportunistic Infections defined a case as "a person who (1) has either biopsy-proven KS or biopsy-proven, life-threatening opportunistic infection, (2) is under age 60, and (3) has no history of either immunosuppressive underlying illness or immunosuppressive therapy."[78] This would later be broadened to include a person having one of several diseases "at least moderately predictive of a defect in cell-mediated immunity, occurring in a person with no known cause for diminished resistance to that disease."[79] The AIDS case definition became progressively more controversial as advocates sought its expansion. Skeptics also argued that a diagnosis of Reye's syndrome was extremely hard to confirm and that many alleged cases were actually something else, thus raising doubt about the validity of epidemiologic studies linking aspirin and Reye's syndrome.[80]

Among the tougher case definition disputes to arise in recent years has been chronic fatigue syndrome. Easily written off as either a tenacious flu or a psychosomatic illness—initially dismissed by many as a new form of yuppie hypochondria—and bearing a diverse array of clinical manifestations, CFS presented a particularly difficult challenge.[81] As Gary Holmes, a CDC staff epidemiologist remarked, many sufferers were described in such vague terms that investigators "couldn't be sure who was a true case and who wasn't."[82] Unlike toxic shock syndrome or AIDS, CFS took years to acquire a distinctive identity; in March 1988 the CDC convened a conference of experts that finally worked out a consensus definition of the syndrome.[83] Unfortunately, the major criteria of the definition consisted essentially of a "new onset of persistent or relapsing, debilitating fatigue or easy fatigability" for which no plausible cause can be found. Hence the disease is defined largely by what it is not. The eleven minor criteria, which include such symptoms as sore throat, mild fever, muscle discomfort, and "unexplained generalized muscle weakness," might be triggered by many other diseases. Even though a case must satisfy the major criteria along with at least six minor criteria, identifying true cases remains difficult.

Case definitions are significant beyond public health agencies and the technical requirements of surveillance. Ill persons crave some explanation, or at least a label, to which they can attribute their afflictions. At the purely psychological level, some persons will find it unsettling to be told that nothing (or nothing identifiable) can be found wrong with them. Others may have problems that, while connected to a recognized ailment, fall just outside the borders of a stringent case definition.[84] Such persons may feel neglected by the scientific or public health establishments, as have DPT parents and many who have suffered from Lyme disease, chronic fatigue syndrome, and the array of symptoms that used to be called AIDS-related complex (ARC).[85] In the AIDS epidemic, the opposite also applies; the disease (and thus its case definition) stigmatizes the infected.

More tangible needs also may exist. With a product-associated illness, a case definition's inclusiveness has major implications for who may seek legal redress. No lawsuit for damages will get far unless a plaintiff can demonstrate, at the very least, that the injury suffered can be plausibly linked with the defendant's product. If monetary or other types of benefits are designated for victims of a particular ailment, these might conceivably be denied to persons who failed to meet a case definition.

In the 1980s difficulties arose in the distribution of social security benefits to some people with AIDS. Trouble could have been expected when the CDC's AIDS case definition was employed by a different agency charged with a different mission.[86] Use of the definition by the Social Security Administration (SSA) led to complaints of unfair treatment for HIV-infected women, who often contracted disabling opportunistic diseases that strict adherence to the CDC definition would exclude. On this basis, SSA failed to list these manifestations of the syndrome among those having a presumptive claim to recognition. This meant that the denied claimants were unable to receive six months of supplemental security income (SSI) benefits on a provisional basis while applying for permanent enrollment in the SSI program. SSA's repeated assertions that it was not bound by the CDC definition did little to placate women's health advocates. They charged that in practice SSA relied on the CDC definition verbatim.[87]

Responses to this situation were predictable. By the early 1990s momentum for change was building through litigation and the legislative process.[88] In 1991 Representative Robert T. Matsui, Democrat of California, and Senators Donald N. Riegle, Jr., Democrat of Michigan, and Daniel Patrick Moynihan, Democrat of New York, proposed legislation intended to generate recommendations for a revised definition of disability. In June 1993 the Clinton administration announced a major relaxation of rules governing the ability of persons with HIV disease to claim disability benefits.[89] Such complications are understandably secondary for those authorities who craft case definitions, for whom the complex and more immediate demands of epidemiologic surveillance and study predominate.

The AIDS definition and surveillance originated without much overt disagreement but proved increasingly controversial as the epidemic matured. Critics argued not only that social security benefits were being unjustly denied but also that the overall research agenda for, and public perception of, the disease has been badly skewed by a continuing identification of AIDS with its manifestations in adult male homosexuals. Moreover, because federal legislation—the Ryan White Comprehensive AIDS Resources Emergency (CARE) Act of 1990—distributed AIDS-targeted grant funds to states and cities according to formulas predicated on local caseloads, subnational governments hungry for assistance had an interest in the scope of the case definition.[90] In November 1991 the CDC proposed to expand its definition beyond the twenty-three AIDS-defining conditions then formally recognized. The agency wanted to include "all HIV-positive persons with CD4+ lymphocyte counts below 200 cells/mm^3[,] . . . CD4+ lymphocytes [being] the primary target cell for HIV . . . [and the counts for which are] a recognized marker of the progression of HIV-related immunosuppression."[91] This expansion proved insufficient to satisfy AIDS advocates, and three conditions (pulmonary tuberculosis, recurrent bacterial pneumonia, and invasive cervical cancer) were added to the definition at the start of 1993.[92] Advocates argued that inclusion of more opportunistic conditions in AIDS surveillance would offer a better picture of the epidemic's evolving impact on women and injection drug users.

As a public record of governmental and private sector performance builds, and the number of affected persons and institutions increases, the potential also grows for dissatisfaction with past and proposed response. When the CDC reported in 1990 that a young woman may have been infected with HIV by a Florida dentist, the agency's inquiry into the matter became the subject of a congressional investigation.[93] Persistent weaknesses in the data documenting the collective long-term experiences of women with silicone breast implants led to blaming both implant manufacturers for their failure to gather such data and the FDA for failing to require their collection.[94]

The proposed Survey of Health and AIDS Risk Prevalence (SHARP) became a major controversy over information gathering, the result of an unavoidable linkage between AIDS and morality. The National Institute of Child Health and Human Development (NICHD), a part of NIH, proposed to contract with the National Opinion Research Center at the University of Chicago for "a large-scale feasibility study designed to assess how best to gather nationally representative data on adult sexual behavior."[95] If successfully completed, the pretest would lead to a full-scale national survey of health and sexual behavior. Numerous prestigious organizations supported the idea of the survey as the best way to obtain data that would help estimate the extent of behaviors associated with HIV transmission and provide a knowledge base for prediction and planning efforts in the fight against AIDS. The project was also designed to yield information on other sexually transmitted diseases and on the use of contraceptives, deemed by some experts as important to more effective policymaking for unwanted pregnancies.

Despite winning the approval of the NIH director and numerous commentators outside government, the proposed contract sparked an extended political clash involving Congress and the upper reaches of the Bush administration. Liberals in both houses of Congress, citing the support of the National Academy of Sciences among others, urged that the survey be approved.[96] The Senate Appropriations Committee said it was "dismayed that the survey of health and AIDS risk prevalence continues to be delayed, and urges the Department [of Health and Human Services (HHS)] to approve the feasibility phase of SHARP promptly. Upon completion of the pilot study by the NICHD, the Committee requests that the Institute recommend whether to launch the full-scale phase of the study and, if appropriate, to make a specific [budget] request for this."[97]

But the corresponding House committee language reflected a different view, noting tersely that "no funds have been requested by the President or added by the Committee for large-scale survey-type studies regarding sexual behavior and AIDS."[98] The proposed survey also raised the ire of conservative Representative William E. Dannemeyer, Republican of California, who branded it an "Orwellian intrusion into the lives of Americans" prompted not by the threat of AIDS but by the political aspirations of gay activists anxious to demonstrate, at taxpayer expense, that homosexual behavior was more widespread than commonly thought.[99] Reviewers at the Office of Management and Budget (OMB) also balked at some of the questions and got HHS to revise the survey. But these revisions failed to satisfy OMB Director Richard G. Darman, who felt the survey ranged too far beyond AIDS, embracing "the more general subject of sexual mores, preferences, and behavior patterns in American society."[100] At Darman's instigation, HHS Secretary Louis W. Sullivan delayed the survey in April 1989, directing the Public Health Service to "conduct a thorough review and revision" of the survey.[101] With this controversy in mind, HHS officials also blocked funding for an entirely different survey of adolescent sexual behavior by a team of sociologists at the University of North Carolina, a proposal that had won the enthusiastic approval of NIH peer reviewers.

Ultimately, Congress would explicitly kill federal funding for both surveys. The 1993 NIH Revitalization Act explicitly forbids the HHS secretary to support either "the SHARP survey of adult sexual behavior or the American Teenage Study of adolescent sexual behavior."[102] The core emotion behind all this anxiety was well expressed by Ward Cates, then-director of the division of STD/HIV prevention at the CDC's Center for Prevention Services. "Let's face it," Cates said, "sex makes people crazy."[103]

AIDS advocates and public health professionals had been considerably happier with the 1983 resolution to the delicate problem of AIDS case reporting. In that instance, the CDC and those worried about confidentiality (including gay activists, some treating physicians, and local health departments) agreed to the creation of a unique reporting mechanism that satisfactorily disguised the identities of individuals.[104] However, once testing for HIV infection became available, a consensus on reporting requirements proved far harder to forge.

CONTROVERSY OVER RESULTS. Even though investigators have learned of a disease's existence and mobilized to learn more, there is no guarantee that they will right away grasp even basic facets of the problem at hand. Only in retrospect, for example, did James Todd, the discoverer of toxic shock syndrome, realize that, of the seven cases on which he had based his seminal 1978 article, three were menstruating at the onset of their illness. He had, he admitted, "missed completely the possibility of any connection with tampon use."[105] Determining the relationship between ticks and Lyme arthritis would also take time and research to become established, as would the linkages among sex, blood, and AIDS.

In defense of conclusions based on epidemiologic studies, particularly in the face of intense controversy, officials understandably lean heavily on two related factors: repeated findings and professional consensus. That is, whatever any single study's limitations, its conclusions are more reliable when replicated or tested in further studies; and interpretations reflecting near-universal professional agreement (or at least a modal position within a distribution of opinion) deserve special deference. Such arguments tend to reassure the politicians and political advocates who hear them, unless particularly strong constituent interests or ideology incline them differently.

But where victims are visible, and their advocates organized and unyielding, data and interpretation that minimize risk may be contested.[106] Controversy over the pertussis component of DPT vaccine ignited in 1982, after a local Washington, D.C., television station broadcast a news feature entitled "DPT: Vaccine Roulette" suggesting, with vivid testimonials, a strong connection between the whole-cell pertussis component of DPT vaccine and various adverse neurological outcomes. The report sparked a national scare, the creation of an antivaccine advocacy group (Dissatisfied Parents Together), and new interest in the development of a less dangerous acellular pertussis vaccine. (At the time, only Japan had introduced such a vaccine.) Repeated analysis showing risk to be either extremely low or unproven was cold comfort to parents who believed their children had been injured or placed at undue risk by pertussis vaccine.[107] In short, investigation may spark disagreement to the extent that external observers are primed to downplay or reject its conclusions.[108]

Failure of epidemiologic and laboratory analysis to isolate the cause of disease frustrates the federal and state public health agencies. Should that failure be an intensely public spectacle, the spotlight may turn harsh. Arguably the most dramatic instance of this involved not AIDS (though the period 1981-83 witnessed much anxiety) but Legionnaires' disease. The peculiar nature of the organism helped it evade detection for more than five months, during which the CDC weathered severe criticism. But as CDC Director William Foege would later observe in 1977 Senate testimony, nothing like *Legionella* had ever been found. The overwhelming majority of important disease-causing bacteria then known had been identified before 1920, most of them before the turn of the century.[109] In retrospect, the delay in identifying the cause of the disease does not seem especially blameworthy. A bacterium seemed an unlikely cause. And as Foege noted, the culprit turned out to be "a bacterium that doesn't grow in usual bacteria media or stain with the usual bacterial stains and appears to grow inside cells and perhaps both inside and outside cells. It is . . . fastidious in its dietary habits . . . [and] requires a very narrow pH range for growth."[110]

And yet, in the intense public scrutiny generated by the episode, the CDC found itself attacked, perhaps predictably, for allegedly botching the investigation. Critics charged that, while investigating the illness and deaths among American Legionnaires in the wake of their convention at Philadelphia's Bellevue Stratford Hotel, the CDC had sidetracked a plausible theory: a toxin, not an infectious agent, could be responsible for the disease.[111] (In fact, the agency had considered and largely discarded this possibility.) The CDC was attacked in a congressional hearing, less than four months after the beginning of the outbreak, for failing to pursue all avenues in search of the etiologic agent.[112] The conspicuous failure to isolate the organism in the first weeks after the outbreak, combined with the intensity of the media scrutiny it generated, created an ideal medium for criticism. What is perhaps most striking about the 1976 Legionnaires' disease outbreak is how much was quickly forgotten. Today the episode is often recalled as an unvarnished success story, another feather in the CDC's cap.[113]

In late 1976, however, just the opposite was the case. The investigation generated far more criticism of the CDC than the initial field inquiries into AIDS would.

The nature of the Legionnaires' disease outbreak and response to it were unusual in at least three key respects. First, an extremely condensed scenario was at play with most deaths occurring before the CDC could begin an investigation. The media, and thus the larger public, found out about the outbreak at virtually the same time as the CDC did. Second, intense publicity and scrutiny were directed at the investigation; unprecedented and sustained press coverage erupted simultaneously with official response. These two factors alone might not have turned the episode into a political disaster for the agency. Had the CDC been able to discover and publicly announce the cause quickly in the face of these two forces, victory might have tasted all the sweeter. However, a third element, an unusual microbe, proved disastrous. The nature of the bacterium helped it elude all efforts to discern its existence until more than five months after the outbreak had started when Joseph McDade and Charles Shepard of the CDC staff, almost by accident, found the *Legionella* and confirmed its relationship to the mysterious outbreak.[114] But by then, the episode had damaged the agency's image. The overlap with the swine flu affair, which directly precipitated Sencer's dismissal as CDC director, was particularly unfortunate.[115]

Conclusion

If detecting and investigating epidemics are not always easy jobs, neither are they usually ripe for controversy unless a problem drags on. If that happens, politicians, organized interests, and the press may challenge the inquiry. For most epidemics, however, this is extremely unlikely. The episode is over too quickly, and no aggrieved constituency is mobilized. Curious journalists soon move on to other topics. To the extent that the CDC and the FDA are slow to detect a problem, they are unlikely to incur significant political blame unless they fail to mount a prompt, serious investigative response once a likely hazard emerges. This is an avoidable trap.

Sometimes, dissatisfaction with CDC or FDA performance arises for reasons the agencies do not control and cannot easily or quickly overcome. Officials can do little to assure that hazards always arise in starkly perceivable clusters, that no manufacturer is ever inclined to hide data, that every new problem will resemble familiar ones, or that epidemiologic inquiry will not spill over into non-health-related issues such as equity and morality. Lyme disease did not begin as a particularly controversial disease, but intense public disagreement would eventually arise over whether the ailment was being underdiagnosed or overdiagnosed, a quandary for which no simple solution was apparent.[116]

In contrast to the Legionnaires' disease imbroglio, the primary political fallout from a continuing inability to isolate a causal agent for chronic fatigue syndrome has been increased research resources through the NIH instead of political attacks on the CDC.[117] But CFS appeared as a relatively undramatic new ailment. Given a cluster of deaths and an avalanche of press coverage, response to the disease would have developed much differently. Even for AIDS, a befuddling and deadly epidemiologic problem from the outset, field investigation and surveillance were not initially politicized. That would occur later. The first year of the recognized epidemic (roughly spring 1981 to spring 1982) produced but a single congressional hearing noteworthy for its gentle treatment of the CDC despite failures of detection.[118] Instead, House Energy and Commerce Subcommittee on Health and the Environment Chairman Henry Waxman concentrated on generating more elite and public attention for the disease and on castigating the Reagan administration for cuts in the federal health budget.[119] By 1983, however, an argument had erupted over the conditions under which a congressional subcommittee would have access to sensitive CDC surveillance files—a fight about institutional prerogatives.[120] And as an ongoing epidemic with very high mortality, AIDS would raise continuing controversy over the size and likely future course of victimization. By the end of the 1980s HIV disease in the United States seemed to have spread significantly through heterosexual contact mainly in low-income urban neighborhoods. Many gay men, at least those who were older and in high-prevalence areas, seemed to be protecting themselves effectively.[121] Was the epidemic increasing, stable, or in decline?[122]

In the case of swine flu, controversy would spring not from problems in discovery or initial inquiry but from what turned out to be an erroneous intervention decision. Only a few weeks elapsed between outbreak discovery and presidential announcement of a massive ill-fated policy response—a national vaccination program. The threat had been posed during a presidential election year as an imminent public health emergency having a distant but frightening precedent in the 1918-19 epidemic. The possibility that the hazard could produce many thousands of very visible deaths cutting across all political and class boundaries helped make expedited response irresistible.[123] Field investigation and related laboratory analysis did not appear especially problematic.

Four

Interventions

To control and contain disease, public health agencies must intervene among specific individuals immediately affected and exercise a broader preventive influence through education and advice. The two activities are strongly interrelated. For neither task can public health agencies assume cooperation from health professionals, business firms, other arms of government, or the general public. Both tasks are more likely than outbreak investigation to prove politically problematic in ways that federal health officials cannot control.

Common-source epidemics of acute disease require the least troublesome intervention, especially when business firms are cooperative and the public education task relatively simple. When certain brands of infant formula and L-tryptophan triggered disease outbreaks, manufacturers were successfully pressured to withdraw the product from the market (although recall compliance was not immediately complete) and consumers were advised not to use the products. A restaurant chain's sale of contaminated hamburger, which led to hundreds of confirmed reports of infection with *E. coli* 057:H7 in the northwestern United States, created a similar situation.[1] The message intended to modify consumer behavior was simple, direct, and powerful: Do not consume or you may get very sick, very soon. Those hearing the cautionary message were not vitally dependent on, or addicted to, the damaging product, and once companies had effectively withdrawn it, continued consumer attention was not necessary. Similarly, a cholera-contaminated well or building cooling system harboring the *Legionella* organism places the main compliance burden on a discrete institution or location. Politicians, the press, and the public would justifiably expect on-site action grounded in sanitary engineering to succeed rapidly.

But matters are sometimes more complicated, technically and politically. A central technical issue is the reliability of field intervention

58

tools. A public health problem becomes inherently more difficult to address as (1) the scope of mass action, or reaction, required increases, and (2) the complexity or required reliability of the intervention technology, such as education or immunization, escalates. As a general rule, people are harder to find and to control over time than places—and the more of either, the tougher the problem. To the extent that intervention must make available, and inspire acceptance of, preventive or treatment regimens, imperfect choices result.

Intervention also has political elements. Officials must allocate resources and decide strategy. Even if they focus carefully on a problem, disagreement may occur over the level and distribution of resources and over the efficacy or ethics of intervention strategies. Once again public health authorities find their jobs complicated as they must face issues beyond disease containment and prevention. Rights, morality, and economic interests may impede consensus on intervention policymaking. Politicians, interest groups, and public sentiment constrain the available options at every level of government.

Public health authorities have at least four traditional tactics for intervening among individuals: (1) restrictions on free movement; (2) case finding, often through testing; (3) distribution of vaccines and therapies; and (4) preventive advice.[2] Ideally, the variety of responses to an emergency interact to form an overall strategy. Effective case finding and vaccine and therapy distribution may hinge on public awareness and acceptance. Case finding is essential to education when people are to receive counseling about future risks, recommended behavior, or therapeutic options. Where a lack of technological innovation renders vaccines and therapies either highly imperfect or altogether unavailable, education becomes a paramount intervention. However pursued, individual awareness has proved both a vital and troublesome component of virtually every disease control campaign.

Government tactics rely heavily on three types of resources: (1) information, backed by suasion; (2) mandates and restrictions; and (3) money and personnel. Information includes data, experience, and interpretive expertise made available through such methods as intragovernmental and intergovernmental consultation, contacts between ordinary citizens and health providers, publicity through the media, product labeling, and telephone hot lines. Health agencies disseminate information to the public and to health professionals. Absent other resources, however, information in any form is mere advice. Mandates and restrictions denote things that government officials and professionals must either do or avoid doing. And all tactics and resources depend on allocations of funds and staff sufficient to implement them.

Federal Capacity and Emergent Public Health Hazards

The menu of realistic and dependably efficacious responses to emergent public health hazards is limited. As is often true, disagreement and institutional fragmentation result in delay and weakened policies. AIDS proved especially difficult, repeatedly pitting public health imperatives against traditional moral beliefs, widespread squeamishness about frank discussion of sex, and anxiety about individual rights. And a lack of careful evaluation has often hindered knowing how well AIDS interventions work.

Restricting Personal Movement

In everyday usage, *quarantine* means "the establishing of a boundary to separate the contaminated from the uncontaminated."[3] Throughout the history of communicable disease, the healthy have been strongly inclined to flee or incarcerate the sick, a tendency that acquired official legitimacy as far back as the Middle Ages when the church devised elaborate rituals to shut lepers out of mainstream society.[4] As recently as the 1940s the TB sanatorium, where patients could partake of fresh air and communal life apart from their uninfected fellow citizens, was an accepted part of the national landscape.[5] The discovery of effective antibiotic treatment spelled the end of the TB sanatorium.[6]

Although state and local health officials can still restrict personal movement coercively, this is rarely necessary because of vaccines, antibiotics, and modern sanitation. As a recent volume on public health law said:

Although modern epidemiology appears to rely on exclusion of cases and contacts from school or work to a far greater extent than on the more extreme measures of isolation and quarantine, the laws of the 50 states go far in authorizing more stringent methods of control than are generally applied in modern practice. With the worldwide eradication of smallpox, the last disease for which strict quarantine, in the old use of the term, was recommended, there seems to be little need for this authority. However, laws in all states still authorize quarantine for a large number of the common communicable diseases.[7]

The federal government likewise retains authority to limit the movement of stricken individuals. Department of Health and Human Services regulations stipulate that "a person who has a communicable disease in the communicable period shall not travel from one State or possession to another without a permit from the health officer of the State, possession or locality of destination, if such permit is required under the law applicable to the place of destination."[8] The regulations give the government authority over the movements of persons with cholera, plague, smallpox, typhus, or yellow fever, who are required to apply for a federal permit for interstate travel.[9]

But the federal regulations promise little or no practical benefit today. The surgeon general, who was removed as head of the PHS in the 1960s, no longer holds the significant authority indicated in the provisions. Furthermore, medical advances have made the regulations largely moot. Smallpox is officially eradicated. The last indigenous and imported cases of yellow fever appeared in the United States in 1911 and 1924, respectively.[10] (And humans contract it only from the bite of certain mosquitoes, not from one another.) For all its historical resonance as the fourteenth century's Black Death, bubonic plague is now preventable through vaccine, treatable with antibiotics, and extremely rare. (Fewer than twenty cases are reported most years.) Murine typhus, transmitted by fleas, claims fewer than one hundred reported victims annually. And the practical constraints attending any genuine enforcement effort must be considered. Who would check the permits? How would one proceed against violators? The provisions generate no controversy because they are not used.

Federal regulations also give the CDC authority to "detain, isolate, or place . . . under surveillance" any person arriving in a U.S. port of entry who "is infected with or has been exposed to" cholera, diphtheria, infectious tuberculosis, plague, suspected smallpox, yellow fever, or suspected viral hemorrhagic fevers.[11] This list, much reduced from a pre-1985 version, reflects a broad professional consensus regarding the diminished benefit of such restrictions in disease control.[12] The agency's division of quarantine currently operates eight quarantine stations (down from some fifty-five in the late 1960s) and otherwise relies mostly on immigration and customs personnel to check passengers and crews for obvious signs of communicable disease at ports of entry, with potential carriers referred to CDC field staff for further inquiry.[13] An Institute of Medicine committee noted in 1992 that the CDC power to detain and isolate individuals had only been invoked three times in the preceding decade.[14] And a new or previously unrecognized ailment cannot, by definition, be placed on any list.

But national policy cannot wholly dismiss restricted freedom of movement as either an absurdity or historical curiosity. Smallpox may pose no threat but the listing of most diseases reflects conscious anticipatory caution.[15] Cholera is rare in the United States, but a massive South American outbreak in the early 1990s confirms its continuing seriousness.[16] (In February 1992 some thirty-one passengers on a Los Angeles-bound flight from Buenos Aires were found to have cholera.)[17] Human cases of plague also are rare in the United States, but viral reservoirs remain both abroad and in the squirrel and rodent populations of the American West. In pneumonic form, plague can spread among humans and can be fatal unless quickly treated.[18] Most fearsome are the viral hemorrhagic fevers (such as Lassa, Marburg, and Ebola), arguably the deadliest of the known communicable diseases. (They are so dangerous that only two laboratories in the United States are equipped to handle them.)[19] Having such hazards on a short list of proscribed diseases will not keep them out but remains a relatively low-cost and direct approach to vigilance.

A stronger rationale for restricted personal movement lies in tuberculosis, AIDS, and the "alliance of terror" between them.[20] A resurgence in TB cases since the mid-1980s, accompanied by a new proliferation of drug-resistant strains of the TB bacillus, has helped renew a cautious interest in imposing restrictions.[21] Active TB is a serious and highly infectious respiratory ailment, particularly among persons with the depressed immune systems characteristic of advanced HIV disease. From 1990 to mid-1992, federal, state, and local authorities collaborated in the investigation of eight institutional outbreaks of multidrug-resistant tuberculosis (MDR-TB) in hospitals and correctional facilities—outbreaks accounting for a total of 236 cases of MDR-TB and fatality rates of well above 50 percent.[22] Most of these patients were HIV-infected, and virtually all harbored organisms resistant to isoniazid and rifampin, the two premier antituberculosis drugs. (Some organisms displayed resistance to as many as seven drugs.) A deadly synergy links HIV and TB; patients with the former are prone to the latter, and TB helps to precipitate full-blown AIDS.[23]

Because social disorganization—reflected in, for example, poverty, homelessness, drug abuse, and mental illness—is common among TB patients, and because successful treatment of the disease requires months of intensive drug therapy, patient compliance is uneven. And if therapy is incomplete, the disease may recur. Patients may also develop MDR-TB organisms from irregular compliance, and these are transmissible to others in close quarters. Despite Americans' customary hypersensitivity to civil liberties, a federal task force recommended the management of noncompliant patients through "a continuum of approaches," with involuntary detention a last resort. A draft recommendation to the states prepared under CDC auspices counsels that "patients who are nonadherent with self-administered therapy should be ordered to continue their treatment under directly observed therapy (DOT) at the direction of the health care provider or other responsible person. If a patient remains infectious while on treatment, states should require the isolation of that individual to protect the public."[24] In early 1993 the New York City department of health did just that, adopting tough new regulations for detaining recalcitrant TB patients throughout their course of treatment instead of, as previously, only for the first weeks until they are noncontagious.[25] According to a survey by Ronald Bayer of the Columbia University School of Public Health, some four hundred persons were "institutionalized on a compulsory basis because of their failure to comply with tuberculosis control requirements" between 1981 and 1990.[26] This contrasts with very few instances of isolation to prevent HIV transmission, and then only in states where very low AIDS counts (and relatively weak AIDS political advocacy) made the policy feasible.[27]

MDR-TB presents a challenge both ironic and severe. It is ironic that the disease is more likely in persons having prior (albeit incompletely curative) drug therapy.[28] It is severe because of both high mortality and the dilemma posed by those incurable patients who do not die. One study concluded with a grim social prognosis:

Fully 46 percent of our patients with treatment failure or relapses died. Physicians and society must recognize that multidrug-resistant tuberculosis is an ominous, deadly disease.

Patients who are treated unsuccessfully but remain alive pose a major public health problem. They must be isolated because of the risk of transmitting virtually untreatable drug-resistant disease. . . . Because of their prolonged shedding of tubercle bacilli, previously treated patients with drug resistance had higher numbers of tuberculin-positive contacts than patients without resistance. . . . Quarantine of patients with treatment failure in their homes is a potential remedy but is seldom achievable. Confinement of patients may protect others, but they must then bear the additional burdens of isolation and stigmatization.[29]

Coercive detention for TB case management, a potential magnet for civil liberties concerns, provoked little overt disagreement during the late 1980s and early 1990s as caseloads rose. Detention was rarely imposed, and no resourceful challenge by anyone claiming undue victimization by government authorities had inspired the assistance of politicians, the press, or a sympathetic court.[30]

The HIV epidemic also led to immigration and travel restrictions in 1987, triggering a long-running controversy that became especially intense nearly three years later, when the detention of an HIV-positive AIDS educator from Holland threatened to disrupt the sixth international conference on AIDS scheduled for San Francisco.[31] Immigration law has long provided for the exclusion of persons with certain communicable diseases, and a 1987 PHS rule made HIV infection one of eight conditions subject to exclusion. The policy has precipitated an ongoing boycott by planners of the annual international AIDS conference, which has since been held outside the United States even though HIV-positive conference attendees would be eligible for a waiver allowing them to enter the country temporarily.

During the 1993 debate on NIH reauthorization, Congress voted overwhelmingly to codify the ban in legislation, a rejection of President Bill Clinton's pledge to reverse it through administrative action. Even some liberal Democrats (along with the New York Times) supported the ban, largely because of anxiety about health care costs and partly because of a widespread sense that the implications of a reversal had been insufficiently studied. (The legislation provided for study.)[32] Critics argued that the measure did not reflect a consensus among public health professionals and that the CDC had previously recommended that the list of "excludable conditions" be reduced to infectious TB only.[33] Many public health experts and AIDS activists were predictably outraged. Lawrence O. Gostin, professor of health law at the Harvard School of Public Health, complained that the ban was misplaced, saying it would neither "reduce the reservoir of infection in the world" nor "provide more resources for counseling and education."[34] Both Gostin and John S. James, editor and publisher of the *AIDS Treatment News*, suggested that the United States had almost certainly exported far more HIV than it had imported over the years.[35] Nevertheless, rising concern about health care costs and an understandable desire to thwart any controllable source of HIV led Congress to choose a more cautious policy.[36]

Testing and the HIV Epidemic

Intervention against many diseases has relied on case finding. On a compulsory or voluntary basis, authorities may want to locate individuals with specific conditions, then use the information they derive to help locate and treat still others with the same condition or at risk of developing it. Assuming a reliable diagnostic test exists for a given condition (an important and not always valid assumption), a central determination must be made regarding how extensive and stringent any testing or screening regime should be.

A number of questions then arise: What happens to the person tested and to others identified as possibly infected in the wake of a positive result? More explicitly, what counsel or treatment ought persons testing positive and their contacts to receive? Will these be provided? What legal or administrative actions are appropriate? What can and should be done to ensure confidential test results? A different concern is preventing wasteful testing. Persons facing little risk (the "worried well") may seek testing (and perhaps even treatment) to address their fears. And fearful politicians may urge testing low-prevalence populations— an approach yielding few cases, a high cost per case identified, and many false positives.

Counting cases is difficult but not usually controversial. Nor, in most instances, does case finding for purposes of treatment and prevention pose many nonmedical worries.[37] When disease advocates and scientists alike bemoan the lack of good tests to detect the Lyme spirochete, the main concern is that false negatives will go untreated, not that persons testing positive will be mistreated.[38] The person with Lyme disease, which is not contagious, bears no social stigma.[39] Much the same would hold for a product-associated illness such as toxic shock syndrome triggered by tampons or pelvic inflammatory disease among Dalkon Shield wearers. Even persons with influenza, a readily transmissible ailment, are spared social opprobrium. Because most infectious diseases prompt a relatively benign social response toward the infected, worries about discrimination against those who test positive or about unwarranted invasions of their privacy tend to be manageable.

However, some infectious conditions may stigmatize. AIDS is the paramount example today as was leprosy a millenium ago. AIDS in the United States has been concentrated in already stigmatized groups and shows every sign of continuing to do so.[40]

Not surprisingly, testing, contact tracing, partner notification, and detailed case reporting for the HIV epidemic have proven persistently controversial, especially in high-prevalence locales.[41] Controversy over AIDS case reporting abated with the creation of a system offering strong protections for confidentiality. Reporting HIV infection has proved a more difficult problem, despite the view of many public health officials that, given voluntary testing and strong procedural safeguards of confidentiality, this traditional public health tool ought consistently to be part of the anti-AIDS repertoire.[42]

Though an AIDS diagnosis had become a reportable condition in every state by 1983, controversy over testing would not erupt until the licensing of an antibody test, the enzyme linked immunosorbent assay (ELISA) in 1985.[43] The dispute is well summarized in a National Research Council study, *The Social Impact of AIDS in the United States*:

> Controversy centered on the role of testing in supporting the radical modifications of behavior that were universally deemed to be critical to altering the epidemic's course. Proponents of aggressive but voluntary testing believed that knowledge of HIV status could be an important motivator of behavioral change, but gay leaders and their allies were skeptical. They suggested that the required changes could best be produced by aggressive education and by appropriately targeted strategies of individualized counseling even if individuals did not know their status. This debate was framed by the fears of gay men and those who spoke on their behalf that the putative benefits that testing could produce could not outweigh the negative psychological and social consequences of being identified as

infected—loss of jobs, insurance, and housing. "Don't take the test" became their rallying cry.[44]

In 1985 CDC Director James Mason suggested that public health departments might maintain records of persons identified by the test as HIV infected and perhaps, given appropriate safeguards, require testing.[45] Other sexually transmitted diseases had been addressed through a "sensitive confidential system" that "doesn't have to be rearranged or reworked to serve equally well in the control of AIDS," argued Mason. Gay organizations disagreed vehemently, contending that because no treatment could be offered persons identified with HIV, persons at risk would have little incentive to cooperate with a testing regime. Coercive testing, the argument ran, might drive the epidemic underground. The AIDS Action Council and the National Gay Task Force advocated anonymous, voluntary testing, believing that compliance depended on such conditions.

Some state and local health officials were similarly wary of testing for political reasons. As Ronald Bayer pointed out, the crucial constraint was a health official's local constituency. The more AIDS cases in an official's domain, the less likely aggressive testing and reporting would be considered or openly supported. A heavy AIDS caseload meant that the official would seek "to preserve collaborative working relationships with relatively large and well-organized gay communities [and remain sensitive to] how reporting would affect the willingness of individuals to be tested."[46] Few AIDS cases would leave the official free to embrace tough traditional measures.

Faced with this situation, the CDC had to tread carefully. In March 1986 the agency's published recommendations on voluntary testing programs cautiously urged that "state and local health officials should evaluate the implications of requiring the reporting of repeatedly reactive . . . antibody test results to the state health department."[47]

In some low-prevalence jurisdictions, health officials adopted, in the face of sometimes intense resistance, a more traditional public health approach.[48] In November 1985 the Colorado State Board of Health unanimously added HIV to the list of more than fifty infectious disease diagnostic test results that clinical laboratories had to report.[49] Regulation of gay bathhouses and provisions for restraining recalcitrant infected persons ensued; though controversial, these triggered far less rancor than similar debates in the AIDS epicenters of New York and

San Francisco.[50] The Minnesota Department of Health, which had logged only 840 cumulative AIDS cases by 1990, pursued aggressive testing, named reporting and contact tracing, and engaged in a well-publicized confrontation with a local clinic accused of subverting the state's policy against anonymous testing.[51] The advent of azidothymidine (AZT) in 1987–88, the first antiviral drug approved for use against HIV, markedly changed the climate in which testing was debated, giving public health authorities an important additional and traditional rationale for testing; for the first time, a positive test result offered the possibility of hastening effective treatment.[52]

Contact tracing and partner notification likewise alarmed gay activists when the CDC proposed them in the mid-1980s.[53] Gay organizations viewed both as potential threats to privacy, unmollified by official claims that such programs had an excellent record of confidentiality. Jeffrey Levi of the National Gay Task Force protested to the CDC that "[contact notification], second only to mandatory reporting, has the greatest likelihood of scaring people away from being tested" and could encourage anonymous sex. HIV's long latency period (unlike the classic sexually transmitted diseases), combined with the number and anonymity of sexual contacts among infected individuals, also poses severe challenges to any tracing and notification scheme.[54] Opponents also feared that contact tracing, as a notoriously labor-intensive public health approach, would siphon scarce resources away from the gay community's preferred intervention strategy of preventive education.

As with HIV testing, the strongest state and local support for contact tracing and notification emerged in relatively low-prevalence areas. After much reworking to allay gay community fears, Minnesota announced in 1986 a contact notification program that gave primary emphasis to private notification (or what the CDC called patient referral) as opposed to provider or governmental referral.[55] By 1988 "the majority of states notif[ied] partners of HIV-infected persons upon the request of the infected person," with some fifteen states encouraging "the index person to have health providers notify his or her partner."[56] But only two states, Colorado and Idaho, had developed "active HIV contact tracing programs with specialized staff and resources to trace all named contacts, not just the present partners of infected individuals."[57] Inherent limitations of contact tracing are apparent in the following American Public Health Association summary of the early Colorado experience:

Colorado began HIV contact tracing in 1986 through its STD case investigators. That program is now supported through resources from the state and federal government. Contacts named by index cases are within the most recent months, and follow-up HIV antibody testing is available. From January 1986 to June 1988, the Colorado program had traced 677 contacts of 418 HIV-infected persons. Seventy-two percent of named contacts were notified, and 7 per cent (52) of all named contacts were found to be HIV-infected. Approximately 3 per cent of all persons testing positive for HIV in Colorado were found through the contact tracing program.[58]

The CDC continued to view testing, contact tracing, and notification as valid components of an overall approach to the HIV epidemic, worthy of federal support, albeit with considerable flexibility for state and local health departments. In this view, a positive test result could facilitate individualized counseling and notification (to be followed, perhaps, by another test of the person notified, more counseling and notification, and so on).[59] In 1988 the agency began requiring partner notification, through either patient referral or provider referral, as a condition for state and local health departments to receive federal HIV prevention funds.[60] In fiscal year 1992 the CDC awarded approximately $102.7 million in HIV prevention cooperative agreement funds to support state and local counseling, testing, and partner notification activities.[61] Annual HIV tests on individuals (as opposed to blood donations) increased from about 79,000 in 1985, the first year of test availability, to some 1.2 million by 1989, an increase the agency saw as "directly related to expansion of counseling and testing services into confidential testing sites."[62]

While the CDC had to employ a combination of funding and suasion during the 1980s to entice the cooperation of health departments, providers, and advocacy groups for programs grounded in voluntary testing, some federal institutions successfully insisted on HIV screening of their own personnel without facing comparable political burdens. Secretary of Defense Caspar N. Weinberger decided in October 1985 that his department would test all active-duty personnel, recruits, and reservists for HIV.[63] (By August 1989 the military services had screened 2.1 million of 2.2 million active-duty members and identified some sixty-two hundred HIV-infected persons.)[64] In November 1986 the State Department declared that it would test all foreign service officers, applicants for appointment, and dependents, an announcement followed the next month by the creation of a Labor Department effort to screen all Job Corps students, applicants, and staff.[65] The Weinberger policy was far more expansive than that recommended by the Defense Department's epidemiological board, which had supported the rejection of HIV-positive recruits but dismissed screening of all active-duty personnel as unnecessary.[66] Both the Defense and State Department decisions reflected fear that conditions in the field might uncontrollably expose the uninfected, that live virus vaccines routinely administered to such personnel for overseas duty could pose health risks to infected persons, and that the infected might prove unable to carry out their assigned duties and become, in the end, a financial burden to the government. The Job Corps testing stemmed from anxiety about injection drug users admitted to the program and their potential impact on uninfected participants.[67] The mandatory testing undertaken by these organizations was controversial, but opponents were in much weaker positions than in the high-prevalence locales where such testing was most effectively resisted.

Reagan administration conservatives such as Education Secretary William J. Bennett and White House aide Gary Bauer viewed mass testing more sympathetically than did either the CDC or the surgeon general.[68] President Reagan strongly endorsed mandatory testing of selected groups (such as prison inmates) and routine (if not mandatory) testing of applicants for marriage licenses in his long-awaited maiden statement on the AIDS epidemic in May 1987, a clear defeat for public health officials, most visibly Surgeon General Koop.[69]

While the public health community's emphasis on voluntary testing stemmed from a need to reassure and entice cooperation from those most at risk, conservative fondness for mandatory testing reflected the anxieties of a far broader audience and the impression that they were being downplayed through undue responsiveness to organized homosexuals. A Gallup survey conducted just after Reagan's address found overwhelming public support for the mandatory testing of immigrants, prisoners, and marriage license applicants, with a bare majority inclined toward universal testing.[70] As a result, many elected politicians (again, especially those representing low-prevalence constituencies) embraced mandatory testing initiatives of various kinds. At the federal level, for example, archconservative Representative William Dannemeyer unsuccessfully championed the testing of everyone entering or exiting prison.[71] The Illinois and Louisiana legislatures enacted premarital HIV screening laws, only to repeal them later because of their high cost and the minuscule number of infections detected.[72]

Interest in these now-discredited efforts highlights the potential difficulty of crafting a reasonably balanced policy in an atmosphere of mass anxiety about a new and deadly threat. Fear among the worried well did not stem solely from conservative homophobia. News of HIV infection among celebrities such as actor Rock Hudson and tennis star Arthur Ashe highlighted the disease, reminding the general public that 'AIDS is everybody's problem' and spurring increases in anonymous testing.[73] But these revelations have also wasted resources. In November 1991 basketball superstar Earvin "Magic" Johnson revealed that he had tested positive for HIV, triggering a sudden and sharp national surge in the number of persons seeking testing.[74] Denver public health officials reported that in the twenty working days following the announcement the clientele at that city's HIV counseling and testing site more than tripled over the same period in the previous year. Unfortunately, officials also noted a 279 percent increase in testing of "heterosexuals with no identified risk for HIV infection."[75] In low-prevalence jurisdictions, such as Orange County in California, these spurts in testing tend to yield few additional cases of HIV infection, while imposing a severely (if temporarily) increased burden on local public health resources.[76] Within weeks after Johnson's announcement, local health authorities in California announced that their testing and counseling budgets were facing exhaustion.[77]

Driven by such worries, and the media attention lavished on one young woman with AIDS, the issue of mandatory HIV testing for health care workers took center stage in 1991. The previous year, the CDC had reported that a Florida dentist who had died had apparently infected a patient during an invasive dental procedure.[78] (The dentist was later identified as Dr. David Acer, the patient Kimberly Bergalis.) Late in 1990 the Johns Hopkins Hospital in Baltimore announced that a staff surgeon had died of AIDS, that it had launched a study of eighteen hundred of his former patients (who were to be offered free HIV testing) to determine whether any may have become infected through surgery, and that it wanted new federal guidelines on how hospitals should handle HIV-infected health care workers.[79] By January 1991 the CDC had tentatively attributed two additional cases of apparent HIV transmission to Acer and announced a meeting the following month "to review current information on risks of transmission of HIV and HBV [hepatitis B virus] to patients during invasive procedures and to assess the implications of these risks."[80]

These developments set the stage for an extended clash over whether HIV-infected health care workers were obliged to tell patients of their condition and whether the law should require the testing of such workers.[81] The debate posed questions of immediate relevance to as many as seven thousand HIV-infected physicians who might find their careers severely circumscribed, if not terminated, particularly in light of polling data showing that two of every three patients were inclined to sever a treatment relationship with an infected health care worker.[82]

A coalition of practitioners, AIDS activists, and public health officials argued that voluntary, not mandatory, HIV testing of health care workers was appropriate, emphasizing the far greater possibility of patient-to-worker transmission.[83] The CDC offered a rough guess that somewhere between 13 and 128 Americans might have contracted HIV from a physician or dentist in the decade since the epidemic had been first recognized.[84] Was this a reasonable estimate, and if so, was mandatory testing worth the cost? Given the sketchiness of the data on which the CDC estimate was based, and because the Florida episode was the only verified instance of HIV transmission by a health care worker, many were inclined to answer no on both counts.

And yet the high profile of the issue endured for many months. One factor was mass anxiety about the risk of infection and the belief that patients had a right to know the HIV-status of any health provider performing an invasive procedure.[85] Two major medical associations, the AMA and the American Dental Association, anxious to assuage public fears on behalf of their members, urged infected physicians and dentists either to warn patients of their conditions or to refrain from invasive procedures; providers who believed themselves at risk should have themselves tested.[86] Another factor was Kimberly Bergalis, who, as she was dying of AIDS, made angry statements to the press and spoke before a House committee in support of a mandatory testing bill sponsored by Representative Dannemeyer and named after her.[87]

Predictably, politicians sought policies that would reassure both the general public and the health community. In July 1991 the Senate voted 81 to 18 for a draconian proposal by Senator Jesse Helms, Republican of North Carolina, to mandate ten-year prison sentences and fines up to $10,000 for any HIV-infected health care worker who performed invasive procedures while deliberately keeping the patient unaware of his or her condition.[88] Helms argued that his amendment "does not require mandatory testing and does not apply to emergency situations."[89] But the *Washington Post's* Malcolm Gladwell noted that "although the measure would not explicitly require HIV testing, the assumption of many health care experts is that liability questions created by the bill will force hospitals to require regular testing of their employees."[90] A more moderate proposal with bipartisan leadership support won a unanimous vote the same day.[91] An attempt to combine aggressive action with deference for public health expertise (and thus to defuse support for the Helms proposal), it required states to embrace CDC guidelines issued that week.[92] These recommendations stated flatly that "mandatory testing of . . . [health care workers for HIV and hepatitis] is not recommended. The current assessment of the risk . . . does not support the diversion of resources that would be required to implement mandatory testing programs."[93] The CDC recommended that health care workers "who perform exposure-prone procedures should know their HIV antibody status" and that those infected "should not perform exposure-prone procedures unless they have sought counsel from an expert review panel and been advised [whether and] under what circumstances, if any, they may continue to perform these procedures." Patient notification should be "considered on a case-by-case basis, taking into consideration an assessment of specific risks, confidentiality issues, and available resources."[94]

In the end, a modified version of the Senate leadership proposal, one that mollified health professionals, public health officials, and AIDS activists, became law. In October a House-Senate appropriations conference agreed to language stipulating that "each State Public Health Official shall [within a year] . . . certify to the Secretary of Health and Human Services that . . . [the CDC's guidelines or their equivalent] have been instituted in the State." Compliance would be the responsibility of the state's chief public health officer and had to include "a process for determining what appropriate disciplinary or other actions shall be taken to ensure compliance." Failure could render a state ineligible to receive Public Health Service funds.[95] The provision did not end controversy over health care worker behavior, but it forestalled mandatory testing.

Treatments and Vaccines

The availability of suitable technology supports a third tactic: the distribution of vaccines and therapies. For some diseases, vaccination provided a public health tool bordering on the miraculous. It ended the annual summer scourge of polio and made possible the worldwide eradication of at least one dreaded disease: smallpox.[96] The twentieth century antibiotic revolution profoundly shaped perceptions of microbial disease, rendering it generally much less fearsome.[97]

A primary rationale for aggressive case finding is to convey advice about preventive and therapeutic options and perhaps to deploy an ameliorative technology among individuals. When such a technology exists, the federal government might distribute it directly to patients or physicians (as the CDC does on occasion when shortages occur) but will more commonly either subsidize its delivery by state and local health agencies or recommend its appropriate uses to public and private health providers.[98] Through its sexually transmitted disease, tuberculosis, and immunization funds, the CDC has routinely supported a variety of intervention and health promotion activities.[99] In recent years, the agency has directly subsidized public sector childhood vaccine purchases by state and local health departments.[100] It has also used a large fraction of its total TB elimination budget to support the growing corps of local outreach workers charged with carrying out the months-long DOT efforts among TB patients needed to stem the spread of both drug-susceptible and drug-resistant strains.[101]

Unlike HIV case finding, little controversy has attended these efforts. To the extent that treatment delivery is perceived as routinely effective and occurs through fee-for-service medicine or other private auspices, it is doubly insulated from political oversight and public dispute. This is one reason that Lyme disease has inspired considerable anxiety but relatively muted political controversy. The American Public Health Association (APHA), for example, has been little concerned with the disease. As a nonfatal and noncontagious illness for which available antibiotic therapy was widely deemed generally effective (and whose victims have tended largely to be middle-class or affluent individuals with recourse to private medicine), the disease has been a low priority for the APHA.[102] Another factor has been avoidance of adversarial politics on the part of interest groups, such as the Lyme Disease Foundation, which prefers quiet lobbying.

Should treatment or vaccine distribution by an identifiable institution create its own victims, as was the case during the swine flu debacle of 1976, matters will evolve differently. Such an episode naturally invites the casting of blame, meticulous rehashings of events, and strong challenges to accepted doctrines and processes.[103] A similar dynamic quickly generated anger in the AIDS community over the initial pricing of AZT by Burroughs Wellcome. Even after a 20 percent price reduction by the end of 1987, the drug still cost AIDS patients about $8,000 per year, placing the firm in the difficult position of appearing further to victimize people with AIDS.[104]

Conclusion

When they intervene at the individual level against an emergent hazard, public health officials may be unable to do so reliably and without controversy. Some interventions raise concerns beyond disease control, and some, such as quarantine or detention, fail to do so only because they are employed rarely.

Particularly during the AIDS epidemic, officials have been pressured to balance urgency and restraint, hoping to find and treat the largest possible number of cases without stimulating panic or inflaming prejudice. Congress has been understandably cautious and divided regarding AIDS intervention, torn by competing pressures and anxious to embrace policies that placate attentive interests and the general public. Funding increases aside, however, congressional forays into AIDS policymaking for individual intervention have offered little foreseeable disease control benefit. The number of future HIV infections preventable through restricted immigration is a tiny fraction, at best, of those that will occur otherwise. And because, as of 1994, no instance of patients' acquiring AIDS from a health care worker had been documented beyond six ultimately associated with Dr. Acer, such transmission is apparently extremely rare. The immigration ban and the appropriations mandate for health care workers reflected a legislature that could not avoid taking action, not a legislature with a clear sense of the most effective action to take.

Five

Education

I N PRINCIPLE, education of the public and health professionals is the most pervasively powerful intervention. Appropriately instructed and motivated, individuals can often eliminate hazards and reduce risk. They can learn, for example, how to prepare food to avoid salmonella poisoning and how to avoid or remove the tick that transmits Lyme disease. In the AIDS epidemic, education provided an alternative to aggressive case finding, which raised concerns of privacy, discrimination, and reduced cooperation.

But preventive communication may be difficult to make effective. Childhood immunization requires that parents act only occasionally, and the health message to them might appear a matter of common sense: Get the shots for your child or risk a serious avoidable illness. Yet immunization has often lagged below rates necessary to prevent disease outbreaks, despite efforts to compel compliance through required certification.[1] Health officials also want parents to know that the benefits of immunization vastly outweigh its risks. (In the United States, at least, no significant overall decline in pertussis immunization has occurred traceable to the DPT scare of 1982.)[2] Attempts to counsel parents regarding adverse reactions do not negate the preventive message but inevitably complicate it because the problem of occasionally serious reactions has been widely publicized and can provoke fear.

Some health messages make sustained demands on a target audience for day-to-day vigilance or restraint. To a teenage girl anxious for social acceptance in the short run, the long-term perils of cigarette smoking, crash dieting, or excessive suntanning may seem insignificant. Similarly, advising condom use or sexual abstinence is one thing; inducing consistent, widespread compliance is another. (Ironically, a problem about which little is known may leave society in a kind of blissful ignorance. Because, for example, the cause of chronic fatigue syndrome has not been found, prevention policy cannot be an issue.)

Education of some kind is important for all emergent public health hazards. During "bad batch" episodes and other common-source epidemics, the public must be alerted to products or activities to avoid and preventive routines to implement. A community also must quickly grasp the scope of an epidemic and its attendant symptoms to facilitate treatment and to prevent undue panic. Dispersal of reliable and comprehensible information serves all these purposes. But for some problems, health officials may know neither an accurate message to convey nor how reliably to get targeted individuals to respond. A previously unrecognized infectious agent—for example, the 1976 outbreak of Legionnaires' disease or the earliest recognized clusters of HIV disease in 1980–81—may hinder quick and informed preventive counsel. Field investigation inherently consumes precious time as authorities grope for the situational and behavioral correlates of chronic fatigue syndrome, or toxic shock syndrome, or what looks like a form of arthritis among Connecticut residents.

Political disagreement may also burden preventive instruction. As AIDS, Reye's syndrome, and toxic shock syndrome illustrate, message content may stimulate controversy, especially when economic stakeholders confront significant losses.

AIDS

Uncertainty and controversy bedeviled AIDS education from the beginning.[3] While the sexual and needle-sharing behaviors that transmit HIV have often been successfully modified, the ability to induce change had varied.[4] Many middle- and upper-middle-class homosexual men dramatically altered their sexual practices during the 1980s, the result of collective fear of, and knowledge about, AIDS. "Indeed," wrote Marshall H. Becker and Jill G. Joseph in a frequently quoted assessment, "in some populations of homosexual/bisexual men, this may be the most rapid and profound response to a health threat which has ever been documented."[5] Even the generally less affluent and more disorganized population of injecting drug users was exhibiting significantly modified behavior by the mid-1980s.[6] This included the use of bleach to disinfect needles and syringes.[7]

But behavioral change was neither universal nor always sustained.[8] Gay men in smaller cities continued to engage in anal intercourse without condoms at far higher rates than their brethren in the AIDS epicenters of New York and San Francisco.[9] Younger gay men, in their late teens and early twenties, also proved markedly less inclined to adhere to regimens of "safer sex."[10] A survey in Dallas County, Texas, found that men who had anal sex with men but identified themselves as "straight" were less likely to report consistent condom use; the more "closeted" the individual, the less safe was his behavior.[11] The sexual behavior of large numbers of non-drug-using heterosexuals, both adolescents and adults, has also resisted change.[12] And whatever the short-run effect of "Magic" Johnson's announced infection on the popularity of HIV testing, teens and young adults in a suburban Maryland STD clinic, unlike their elders, displayed no postannouncement inclination to reduce their numbers of sexual partners.[13]

AIDS awareness and prevention information has been widely disseminated over the years through such means as the mass media, posters, and a highly publicized mailing by the surgeon general.[14] But effective instruction must both inform and motivate. Such factors as peer group norms and an individual's sense of efficacy, crucial to motivation, are impossible to influence reliably.[15] Terrifying the target audience is not sufficient because doing so can produce fatalism and denial.[16] When information about the nature and scope of behavior is lacking, informed campaigns of preventive instruction cannot be designed.[17] And all efforts to change behavior—antismoking campaigns and drug and alcohol treatment programs are familiar examples—face the prospect of substantial recidivism.[18]

Complicating the situation has been intense and persistent controversy over the scope and content of AIDS prevention messages.[19] Because HIV disease not only is sexually transmitted but also is associated with sexual promiscuity, homosexual intercourse, and injection drug use, calls for creatively candid preventive education inevitably collided with mainstream moral sensibilities. Moral conservatives, fearful of condoning sexual promiscuity and homosexuality, demanded restrained presentations emphasizing abstinence outside marriage and fidelity within it. AIDS advocates and many health authorities urged frankness, pointing to a rising tally of cases and the futility of inducing the desired change with messages too tepid or vague to work.

The gay community quickly embraced education as its preferred intervention. As Ronald Bayer wrote: "Here was a public health strategy that was utterly compatible with the protection of the private realm, a strategy for the modification of private acts with dire social consequences that did not employ the coercive power of the state."[20] The oft-repeated claim that "the only effective tool we have against AIDS is education" was more political than rigorously factual, a way for the gay community and its allies to fend off calls for increased reliance on testing and reporting. In the throes of a deadly epidemic that simultaneously conjured both public health and civil rights anxieties, the educational option offered activists a positive and politically comfortable disease control agenda.

By the mid-1980s the federal government was struggling to straddle these opposing perspectives. Surgeon General Koop, ironically, found himself battling fellow moral conservatives in the Reagan administration over his pragmatic insistence on preventive instruction that went beyond a pure abstinence-and-fidelity message. The October 1986 surgeon general's report on AIDS dissatisfied persons who were opposed to a purely health-oriented, rather than a moral, approach to AIDS.[21] By 1988, bolstered by an ascending AIDS caseload and congressional support, the Public Health Service was able to mail a six-page brochure entitled "Understanding AIDS: A Message from the Surgeon General" to every household in the country.

CDC funding of local educational initiatives proved politically delicate as well. Its 1986 guidelines for community organizations seeking grants for local education initiatives tried to avoid material that might offend. So the agency required that local program review panels (approved by state and local health officials) oversee grantees.[22] In May 1992 a federal judge struck down this "offensiveness" standard as both inconsistent with the agency's statutory authority and unconstitutionally vague.[23] "Can educational material be offensive simply because it mentions homosexuality?" wrote Judge Shirley Wohl Kram of the U.S. District Court for the Southern District of New York. "Because it depicts an interracial couple? Can a proposed education project be offensive because it traps a captive audience, such as subway riders, and forces them to look at a condom?"[24] AIDS advocates believed some discomfort was inevitable. "There is no way to avoid creating controversy among certain populations," wrote William H. McBeath, executive director of the APHA in commenting to the CDC on proposed program revisions in the wake of the court's decision, "without rendering AIDS prevention educational materials ineffective. Having some of these people on a program review panel . . . is not going to preclude or minimize these controversies." McBeath and others insisted that content review by the panels had a "chilling effect" on AIDS education efforts and was in any case "superfluous" given the origins of such initiatives in the communities to be served.[25]

The CDC also drew fire for lackluster media campaigns.[26] In March 1992, when the agency unveiled its ostensibly improved television, radio, and print media effort (which would eschew mention of the words "sex" or "condom"), the director of education for the American Foundation for AIDS Research reacted with disgust:

> Once again, the Centers for Disease Control have released a public education campaign that is totally oblivious to the lessons AIDS educators have learned the hard way during the first decade of the AIDS epidemic. If the CDC can't level with the American public about condoms and clean needles, our families, friends and neighbors will continue to be reduced to grim statistics.[27]

Such reticence did not originate solely in conservative pressure. The CDC was also unsure how to address diverse populations. Another factor was commercial sensitivity among broadcasters, manifested in a long-standing reluctance to air contraceptive advertising—the overtly sexual content of much commercial programming notwithstanding. As one network representative told a congressional committee in 1987: "A significant portion of our viewers feel contraceptive commercials are inappropriate or offensive, because they appear within or adjacent to programs that they might be viewing with their families, and these commercials appear without warning and out of context."[28] And urban liberals who worried about illegal drug use opposed using federal funds to promote needle cleaning or needle exchange, an innovative intervention.[29] It took a development beyond public health, the election of Bill Clinton, to change the political environment in which AIDS public service announcements were being considered, clearing the way for more aggressive media proselytizing for condom use beginning in 1994.[30]

The CDC has also confronted resistance in advising health care workers (for example, family physicians, surgeons, dentists, nurses) about how to guard against contracting or transmitting HIV. A battle erupted between health professionals and the CDC. While the agency's July 1991 guidelines allowed health advocates to fend off the Helms amendment and mandatory testing, a considerable challenge remained of prompting health care workers to comply with the recommendations. The guidelines said that "exposure-prone procedures" that might place patients at particular risk "should be identified by medical/surgical/ dental organizations and institutions at which the procedures are performed."[31] But many organized health professionals balked.[32] Opponents held such a list scientifically indefensible given the few cases of HIV transmission (all linked to one provider, the Florida dentist) and lingering uncertainty about even those cases.[33] As earlier in 1991, when physician testing and patient notification had been at issue, the AMA leadership focused on reassuring the public, asserting that "ambiguity or uncertainty should be resolved in favor of our patients' interests," a perspective echoed by CDC Director William L. Roper.[34] Faced with a revolt among health care workers, however, both the CDC and the AMA soon capitulated.[35] The agency would emphasize "identifying infected health workers who do not meet standards of infection control or whose stamina or mental state makes them unfit to practice."[36]

Reye's Syndrome

When controversy arose over whether aspirin caused Reye's syndrome, the government faced opposition it could not easily overcome. A CDC official detailed to the Arizona Department of Health Services and several colleagues studied seven school-aged children hospitalized with confirmed cases of RS.[37] All seven had been given aspirin for the flu, while only eight of sixteen controls (also flu victims) had. The RS patients had taken larger doses than had the controls, and more severely ill patients had consumed aspirin in larger amounts. Additional data from Ohio and Michigan appeared to confirm a relationship between RS and aspirin use against the flu.[38] Assuming their validity, the data implied that parents and physicians should receive counseling against using salicylates (that is, aspirin or aspirin-containing products) to reduce fever in children with any flu-like illness. Such a recommendation was bound to prove contentious. Physicians and parents had long resorted to aspirin routinely to reduce fever, and aspirin manufacturers would face potentially severe economic losses.

The CDC quickly understood that methodological ambiguities would provide critics with ammunition. Case-control studies may be subject to recall bias, because of difficulty in obtaining comparable and accurate medication histories for both patients and controls whose memories of even recent illness and behavior may be unreliable. Patients with RS also could have had more severe antecedent illness and thus may have taken more medications, including salicylates, than did matched controls. Or perhaps the infections afflicting cases and controls were not precisely the same. Additional areas of concern to CDC consultants, industry representatives, and others included:

> 1) interviewer bias, i.e., the knowledge of the interviewer of the case-control status of the subject; 2) interview techniques that were not comparable, i.e., medication histories were more often verified (including checking of medication labels) for controls (whose parents were interviewed at home) than for patients (whose parents were usually interviewed in the hospital), which may have resulted in a tendency for parents of patients more often than for parents of controls to misclassify the generic drug used by their children; 3) possible misclassification of Reye syndrome, i.e., since biopsies were not routinely performed, it was possible that some persons with mild illness might be included in the group of patients diagnosed as having Reye syndrome.[39]

As various studies emerged, the aspirin industry aggressively lobbied the CDC and the FDA.[40] CDC Director William Foege believed the association between aspirin use and RS genuine, as did agency consultants who, despite the methodological pitfalls, remained struck by the overall "strength and consistency of the observed association between Reye syndrome and salicylates."[41] The American Academy of Pediatrics committee on infectious diseases agreed.[42]

By early 1982 the Public Citizen Health Research Group (HRG), affiliated with consumer advocate Ralph Nader, had embarked on what would become a lengthy crusade for tougher mandatory warning labels. The HRG petitioned the FDA "to immediately change the labelling on all aspirin-containing products to warn against use by children with chicken pox or during the winter because of the link between aspirin and Reye's Syndrome."[43] The HRG went to court in May 1982 along with the American Public Health Association to try to compel action, a position bolstered the following month by a surgeon general's advisory warning "against the use of salicylate and salicylate-containing medications for children with [influenza and chicken pox]."[44]

The aspirin industry fought the emerging consensus on the RS-aspirin connection. It emphasized methodological concerns and potential adverse effects of aspirin treatment forgone. It also shifted the venue of political combat to more favorable ground. The results were startling. In June 1982 Health and Human Services Secretary Richard S. Schweiker had announced his acceptance of the RS-aspirin connection, directing the FDA to undertake extensive public education in tandem with a required warning label.[45] But by November Schweiker had retreated from this position, saying that any final decision would await a major new government study.[46]

The industry had turned to the regime of regulatory relief imposed by President Reagan in his best known and most widely criticized executive order, number 12291, issued when the administration was barely a month old. The order had granted the Office of Management and Budget unprecedented authority to subject proposed regulations to a cost-benefit test. As writer Tim Miller described:

> After Schweiker announced that he had approved the rule, [Aspirin Foundation] chairman Joseph M. White consulted his attorneys and learned of the O.M.B.'s veto power. He had one more shot to avert the rule. Five foundation representatives met one evening at O.M.B. headquarters with James J. Tozzi, deputy administrator of O.M.B.'s Office of Information and Regulatory Affairs. They gave Tozzi the name of a physician opposed to the label, to whom Tozzi later spoke at length and whose views, Tozzi told me, greatly influenced him.[47]

Shortly thereafter Tozzi would recommend to his boss, Christopher DeMuth, that required labeling be suspended pending further study. DeMuth, in turn, advised Schweiker to reconsider, which the secretary did.

For more than two years thereafter, aspirin makers held their ground, insisting on the results of further study, battling the HRG in court, and publicly downplaying the RS-aspirin connection.[48] A televised proaspirin public service announcement, sponsored by an industry-funded pediatricians' organization, aired on local stations in the fall of 1984. The FDA, the CDC, and Assistant Secretary for Health Edward Brandt all attacked the announcement as misleading.[49]

In January 1985, in the wake of new data from a Public Health Service pilot study showing an RS-aspirin association, Margaret M. Heckler, Schweiker's successor as HHS secretary and a former Republican House member from Massachusetts, called on aspirin makers to offer a voluntary program of public education. In negotiations with the government, the Aspirin Foundation's member companies agreed to a label that made no mention of RS, counseling consumers to "contact a physician before giving this medicine to children, including teenagers, with chicken pox or flu." Meanwhile, the foundation's television ads would state that "although the cause of Reye Syndrome is not known, some studies suggest a possible association with medicines containing salicylate or aspirin. So, it is prudent to consult a doctor before giving these medicines to children or teenagers with chicken pox or flu."[50] The aspirin makers thus continued to evade the strong "do not give" language sought by the HRG and federal public health officials.[51]

By the spring, however, congressional Democrats were prepared to force stronger mandatory labeling. The House Energy and Commerce Subcommittee on Health and the Environment held a March hearing at which Chairman Henry Waxman denounced the voluntary labels as "inadequate and vague" and lacking a "prominent format clearly visible to consumers." They would also appear too late, missing the current flu season. And because Schering-Plough, maker of St. Joseph aspirin for children, was not a member of the Aspirin Foundation, the industry had been incompletely represented in the labeling negotiations.[52] Waxman noted that while "this terrible syndrome is rare"—the National Reye's Syndrome Foundation had reported six child deaths in the first two months of 1985—"even one unnecessary death is too many. . . . If the Department of Health and Human Services can identify risks but is unwilling or unable to take strong enough measures, the Congress must act."[53] He and Senator Howard M. Metzenbaum, Democrat of Ohio, proposed legislation to require labels stating: "WARNING: This product should not be given to individuals under the age of 21 years who have chicken pox, influenza, or flu symptoms. This product contains aspirin or another salicylate which has been strongly associated with the development of Reye's Syndrome, a serious and often fatal childhood disease."[54]

By the end of 1985 congressional Democrats and their consumer allies had won. After ten days of negotiations between the industry and several senators in November, the Aspirin Foundation agreed to a strong mandatory label. The benefits of continued resistance had declined. Child aspirin consumption was down; the voluntary warnings, press coverage, and the availability of a viable substitute product (acetaminophen) had combined to reduce it.[55] The following month the FDA proposed mandatory labeling reading: "WARNING: Children and teenagers should not use this medicine for chicken pox or flu symptoms before a doctor is consulted about Reye's Syndrome, a rare but serious illness."[56] On June 5, 1986, six years after the controversy had erupted, a final regulation became effective. Annual reported cases of RS, which had fallen from a peak of 555 cases in 1980 to approximately 200 cases a year during 1982–84, continued to decline dramatically—to 93 in 1985, 103 in 1986, 36 in 1987 (the first full year in which the mandatory warning regulation was in effect), and 25 cases annually in 1988 and 1989. The precise cause of RS remained unclear, but by the end of the decade few cared. Several years later one study estimated that 1,470 lives could have been saved had the labeling been in place in 1982.[57]

Toxic Shock Syndrome

Labeling for tampons took a remarkably similar course, becoming snared in the machinery of presidential regulatory relief and subject to extended disagreement among manufacturers and consumer groups. A national scare over toxic shock syndrome arose in 1980 with CDC reports of a serious new (though, like RS, apparently rare) disease in menstruating women.[58] Epidemiologic evidence began to implicate tampons as the culprit.[59] But a decade would elapse before an FDA labeling regulation intended to enable women to reduce their risk of developing TSS took effect.

During the winter before the scare, the FDA had designated the tampon as a class II medical device eligible (under the Medical Device Amendments of 1976) for a performance standard.[60] In July 1981 the FDA's Bureau of Medical Devices suggested that the American Society of Testing and Materials (ASTM), a voluntary standards organization, develop a performance standard addressing problems ("broken strings, particulates, cleanliness, shredding, sharp edges, allergies") apart from TSS, about which too little seemed known to permit such an effort.[61] By January 1982 an ASTM tampon task force, which included manufacturer representatives, consumer groups, and the FDA, was operating.[62]

By then, with data strongly implicating tampon absorbency as a key variable in TSS, the government was already warning women to use the minimum absorbency rating necessary to control the menstrual flow.[63] In June 1982 the FDA issued a regulation requiring manufacturers to print this advice on tampon packaging.[64] But because manufacturers did not employ either a standardized absorbency terminology or scale of measurement, women could not easily follow the advice, especially if they wanted to make comparisons across brands. One manufacturer's super tampons might be less absorbent than another's regular. Accordingly, Public Citizen petitioned the FDA in July 1982 to develop "a scientifically and technically justifiable method for measuring the fluid capacity of tampons" along with "a uniform nomenclature" that would be displayed on each package.[65] The agency replied that it was committed to the ASTM task force's deliberations, arguing that "a voluntary standards process is the most efficient and economical method available" for crafting the desired standard.[66]

Two years later the ASTM task force process had broken down, a casualty of irreconcilable priorities and the contrasting market strategies among major manufacturers.[67] While Tambrands, makers of Tampax, wanted descriptive labels ("regular," "super," and "super-plus") indicating a range of absorbency within each label, makers of OB and Playtex tampons defended a single-digit system. Shifting to a range system would obliterate any distinction between products differentiated by number, placing OB and Playtex at a disadvantage.[68] This disagreement would continue into the late 1980s, even after the FDA had responded to the ASTM task force debacle with a pledge to issue its own regulation specifying the absorbency test to be used "with the result to be expressed as a numerical absorbency factor, somewhat analogous to the sun protection factor used in sunscreens."[69]

But for the FDA to write its own regulation would take more time. An advisory committee on obstetric and gynecological devices would have to consider the problem; in August 1985 the committee recommended both absorbency and ingredient labeling.[70] By June 1987 the FDA was preparing a proposal that it submitted, as required by executive order 12291, for OMB review. The FDA proposal stipulated five absorbency ranges, offering acceptable terms (regular, super, and super-plus) to denote the middle three but no terminology for the most and least absorbent classes. The government set October 1987 as the target for issuing a notice of proposed rulemaking. Meanwhile, a new CDC study further solidified the connection between TSS and tampon use, prompting Public Citizen to petition the FDA again, arguing that manufacturers ought "to disclose the actual absorbencies of their products" in lieu of "confusing" descriptive terminology.[71]

In 1987–88, however, OMB delayed the regulation, which the FDA revised (with the ranges intact) and issued in September 1988.[72] But Playtex Family Products continued to object. The proposal would, in the company's view, unacceptably change the absorbency testing system that manufacturers employed and force them "to target absorbency to the middle of each range. As a result those consumers who need to increase absorbency would need to jump from the middle of one range to the middle of the next higher range (about 3 grams). This may be more absorbency than they need." The proposal would also "arbitrarily force Playtex to increase the absorbency of its Super Plus product, which is used by about 1.5 million consumers, by more than 1 full gram." The company claimed it would also have to reduce the absorbency of its regular tampon because of a discrepancy between in vitro and in vivo absorbencies.[73]

The regulatory tussle extended into 1989. Secretive review prevented consumer groups from knowing precisely to what extent OMB was influencing the FDA proposals. The saga ended in October 1989 under court order, as a result of a Public Citizen lawsuit that yielded an August 1989 decision by U.S. District Court Judge Barrington D. Parker assailing FDA rulemaking on tampon labeling as "unreasonably delayed" and setting a deadline of October 30 for promulgation of a final rule.[74] The final rule appeared on October 26 requiring, effective March 1, 1990, five standardized tampon range classes.[75] While gauging the precise health impact of the new rule is difficult, reported cases of TSS declined to 322 in 1990 and 280 in 1991; the 1983–89 average had been 420.[76]

Conclusion

Individual and mass intervention for emergent hazards may be troublesome in ways beyond the easy control of federal officials. An emergent threat that yields identifiable victims in the short run readily claims public attention, but agenda setting is usually the easy part of the problem. Three important complications that officials must cope

with are mass fear, the impact of organized interests, and limited knowledge.

The anxiety that generates political action may work against balanced intervention. Celebrity victims of HIV disease may propel hordes
to descend on testing sites or prompt the creation of premarital screening programs, but with questionable benefits. Though no celebrity with
tuberculosis had stepped forward or been identified, a similar danger
of overuse threatened New York City's TB clinics in the wake of publicity about the resurgence of the disease and the special hazard posed
by drug-resistant strains. One problem with free public clinics,
according to a CDC official detailed to tuberculosis treatment and
prevention in New York City, is that the needs of the acutely ill could
be displaced by the walk-in demands of the worried well.[77] If this is
so, and if the latter are generally more affluent (and hence more likely
to complain effectively when denied acceptable service) than the former, then public attention may undermine well-focused intervention.

As in nearly every other sphere of policymaking, organized interests
defeat or delay policies, notwithstanding the urgency wrought by
immediate victimization and a consensus that intervention or education
is appropriate. Both the RS and TSS episodes would have proven
complex even without OMB involvement and abortive efforts at industry voluntarism that further delayed resolution. (One may speculate
about the extent to which controversy, stimulated by consumer groups
in alliance with politicians and disseminated through the media, might
have had educational benefit independent of the labeling that ultimately resulted. Media coverage can plausibly accomplish some things
better than a label, at least in the short run. The leverage the Natural
Resources Defense Council achieved during the Alar scare is a case in
point.) Policymaking for AIDS education has likewise energized health
care professionals, the blood products industry, and middle-class homosexuals—each an attentive and motivated clientele. AIDS presents not
only a public health disaster but also a civil rights issue, a moral
quandary, and an economic (and, in the health care realm, fiscal) problem. Groups and politicians have had particularly strong incentives to
highlight concerns that a pure public health perspective would deemphasize.

Health education through the mass media arguably falls into a category that economists call "collective goods" such as clean air and
national defense. Such goods or services cannot effectively be provided

to selected members of a community but withheld from others.[78] For the typical health message, maximum dissemination is the ideal; message spillover among those not targeted is unimportant. But an epidemic such as AIDS requires difficult fine-tuning: aggressiveness among targeted populations (gay men and injecting drug users) and restraint for the sake of, say, third graders. Unlike Lyme disease, educational intervention for AIDS was never, and could never have been, solely a question of what works for disease control.

And what works has sometimes remained unclear. The AIDS epidemic had been under way for many years, with preventive education a major recognized concern, without much attention to systematic outcome evaluation.[79] Indeed, organizations delivering health interventions often face institutional disincentives to such evaluations, which redirect scarce resources away from service delivery. The sheer analytical problem also exists of separating program effects from exogenous ones.[80] Investigators learned relatively quickly that many persons at risk of infection could and would change their behavior to reduce the chance of contracting or transmitting the disease. But uncertainty lingered regarding the ability of education campaigns reliably to inspire and sustain the desired behavior, even when such efforts yielded increased knowledge and changed beliefs among targeted groups.[81]

Six

Regulation

R EGULATING THE quality of products and processes is both difficult and controversy-prone for at least three reasons.[1] First, uncertainty abounds. The effect of products approved or withheld, of a change in the way they are monitored or manufactured, or of new market environments is hard to foresee. Second, regulation commands attention. Journalists, judges, politicians, organized policy advocates, and academic observers routinely scrutinize it. Third, regulation incites aggressive and competing responses rooted in ideology, fear, and material self-interest. Claims of underregulation and overregulation resonate widely.

Emergent public health hazards present at least four broad regulatory problems: (1) withdrawing harmful products; (2) avoiding the approval and distribution of harmful products in the first place; (3) hastening product approval where appropriate (for example, fast tracking AIDS drugs); and (4) refining the behavior of industries and professions. Hazardous products are both less and more challenging than communicable diseases. One can remove products, but not infectious diseases, through institutional cooperation. But unlike infectious diseases, products often enjoy business and grassroots constituencies that may fight to ensure their availability. One of the most vexing regulatory problems is the visibly harmful product that cannot reasonably, on account of its demonstrable benefits, be banished.

Product Withdrawals

Although often costly, withdrawals pursue a measurable and easily comprehended goal: retrieval of an offending product from buyers and sellers. A manufacturer or distributor will typically have strong incentives to withdraw acutely hazardous products both to preserve its commercial reputation and to avoid litigation. The FDA also can direct embarrassing media attention to a delinquent business. Moreover, withdrawal often affects only a portion of a company's products. Finally, each manufacturer knows that it may not depend on others to assist in combating a withdrawal because competitors have much to gain from eliminating a bad apple in their midst and much to lose from any perceived support of one.

Notwithstanding such factors, economic incentives do not inevitably incline every business to withdraw a defective product. A company may have many millions of dollars invested in a product or depend heavily on its revenues. Some company executives might calculate that the stakes make resistance or even subterfuge worthwhile, with unacceptable consequences sufficiently unlikely. For this reason, consumer advocates have repeatedly (though so far unsuccessfully) urged Congress to give the FDA unilateral withdrawal authority.[2]

The usually strong incentive for anticipatory withdrawals, and for compliance with those requested, explains why the FDA has been able to function without the formal power to coerce withdrawals. On finding an adulterated product, the agency may request a recall; that is, a "*voluntary* removal or correction of a marketed product that is considered by FDA to violate the [Food, Drug, and Cosmetic Act.]"[3] Or it may initiate a seizure—approaching a U.S. attorney, who files the request in the appropriate federal district court. With court approval, a U.S. marshal may then seize the material.[4] The agency may also seek an injunction against distribution of the product (though some injunctions do order companies to recall products).[5] Or the agency may request the voluntary destruction of the offending product.[6] If a product received FDA approval, the agency may rescind that approval.

Product withdrawal problems fall into two categories. One is the "bad batch," where tampering or failure of quality control creates a hazard. A second is that the product may yield an unacceptable risk/benefit ratio even when correctly constituted and properly used. A tragic example was E-Ferol, an intravenous solution marketed as a vitamin supplement for premature infants in late 1983 and early 1984.[7] The company withdrew it, though not before thirty-two infant deaths had been associated with its use.[8] Premarket approval strives specifically to prevent this situation. (E-Ferol had been marketed without FDA approval.) For both categories, withdrawal is a reasonable option.

But many products offer substantial benefits despite the genuine risks they pose. Products harboring significant risks that nevertheless cannot be banned or easily reformulated lend urgency to labeling and mass education efforts.

Bad Batches

Despite a considerable regulatory apparatus, improperly constituted products appear often, though most consumers are unlikely to encounter any one of them.[9] When such products claim visible victims, publicity is likely and so is a policy response with implications extending beyond the episode at hand.

Two now-distant incidents, and a recent one, are illustrative. In the summer of 1955, seventy-nine recently vaccinated children, and a somewhat larger number of their contacts, contracted poliomyelitis because of an improperly manufactured "killed virus" vaccine (developed by Jonas Salk) from Cutter Laboratories. This outbreak triggered particular fear and debate because the government had just approved the Salk vaccine following successful field trials. Some researchers (most prominently Albert Sabin, developer of the "live" oral vaccine) had challenged the Salk approach as risky and impractical. The so-called Cutter incident led to a reorganization of the Bureau of Biologics, responsible for approving such products.[10] In July 1971 Bon Vivant recalled all its canned foods after botulism-tainted vichyssoise killed a New York man and made his wife seriously ill.[11] Within weeks, the company filed for bankruptcy.[12] The FDA was soon under pressure from consumer activists citing the Bon Vivant episode (and a similar recall prompted by botulism-contaminated Campbell soup that had claimed no victims) as evidence of needed reform. By September the FDA commissioner was before Congress seeking a considerable increase in resources for food plant inspections.[13] More recently, the 1993 outbreak of bloody diarrhea and kidney damage traced to inadequately cooked hamburger prompted reassessment of the national meat inspection system.[14]

The bad batch that claims identifiable victims has a long history of generating legislative and bureaucratic innovation. Repeated expansions in the FDA's legislative mandate have come largely in response to these hazards.[15] A policy status quo (resulting from deadlock, indifference, or satisfaction) yields at least temporarily to a transforming catalytic event—a horror story or crisis. Such events grab the attention of politicians, the media, and policy advocates, altering perceptions of what seems important, defensible, or necessary. They turn problems into issues and expand the "scope of conflict" surrounding existing issues.[16] What looks like adequate, or uninteresting, policy one day can appear inadequate and very interesting the next.

Few members of Congress presumably had given much thought to product tampering before the autumn of 1982, when cyanide-laced Tylenol capsules killed seven people. The national response to this incident was immediate and powerful. The poisonings, the recall, and the subsequent investigation made national headlines.

For all the feverish attention they generated, the poisonings presented a technically and politically manageable problem. The small number of victims, clustered by locale, apparently resulted from a single invidious mind, not a conspiracy or widespread contamination. With no broader hazard to quell, the main problems turned out to be staving off panic and guarding against recurrence. The drug's manufacturer would spend "$300 million to recall 31 million old packages of Tylenol capsules and promote new ones that were 'triple sealed' to resist tampering."[17]

The seven deaths generated political and policy shock waves. The FDA suspended or slowed down lower-priority work to cope with the poisonings.[18] The secretary of health and human services quickly requested the agency to begin work on a new regulation requiring tamper-resistant packaging.[19] The Proprietary Association, representing makers and distributors of nonprescription medications, immediately supported "preemptive Federal Government regulation," which it deemed "essential in order to achieve regulatory uniformity" across the United States.[20] Congress held a hearing barely two weeks after the first death.[21] Within a month, the FDA had ready a new regulation on packaging for most prescription drugs.[22] And within two months, spurred on by copycat tamperings, both the House of Representatives and the Senate had passed antitampering legislation as part of a larger crime bill that subsequently fell victim to a presidential pocket veto for unrelated reasons.[23] Quickly reintroduced and revised in the Ninety-eighth Congress, the Federal Anti-tampering Act became law in October 1983.

This administrative and legislative frenzy shows what is possible when government finds an issue for which attractive policy solutions exist—increased jail terms, larger fines, more effective tamper-resistant packaging—in a context of high public concern, consensus among regulators and regulated interests, and relative scientific certainty. For their part, legislators could construe tampering as a law enforcement problem instead of a scientific one. The political course of the issue could hardly be more different from, for example, clean air debates.

The events of 1982 were also exceptional even among episodes of product tampering. The general problem had been acknowledged at least since the turn of the century, and instances of tampering tied to attempted extortion had occasionally been brought to the attention of the FBI.[24] Since 1982 other cases of tampering have surfaced briefly in the national news media, including another Tylenol homicide in 1986 and a 1991 recall of Sudafed decongestant capsules that caused at least one death.[25] The 1986 Tylenol episode provoked a fresh wave of anxiety and a decision by Johnson & Johnson to abandon the traditional capsule format altogether.[26] But with a law already enacted and a trend toward tamper-evident packaging well under way, no additional policy innovations were forthcoming, though the 1986 poisoning did prompt another congressional hearing—one aimed mostly at educating and reassuring consumers.[27]

The infant formula episode bears similarities.[28] Congressional inquiry into, and criticism of, the FDA's performance led quickly to proposed legislation.[29] The resulting Infant Formula Act, cleared in September 1980, mandated minimum levels of twenty-nine formula nutrients. (The list and nutrient levels were subject to administrative revision.) It formalized record-keeping requirements for formula manufacturers. The new law also mandated administrative action on an infant formula recall regulation and granted explicit authority for, but did not require, a regulation on the quality control procedures employed by manufacturers.

Though the bill progressed through Congress easily, offering an obvious and probably irresistible opportunity for members to claim they were protecting the nation's babies, just how much additional safety the law provided remains unclear. The FDA did not think the legislation was necessary, nor did some key congressional staff who worked on the issue. After all, the law did not target activity that had an overtly supportive constituency; no formula manufacturer who wanted to stay in business would have an incentive to create victims. The FDA did not lack authority to regulate the formula industry. Before the Syntex episode, no recent problem with formula quality had turned up.

Whatever its technical merits, the new law had two practical political effects. It inevitably raised the priority of infant formula as an issue for the FDA. And it would provide fodder for House Democrats attacking the perceived deregulatory excesses of the Reagan administration. When Wyeth Laboratories in 1982 recalled another soy-based formula after company tests indicated a deficiency in vitamin B$_6$, Representatives Al Gore, Democrat of Tennessee, and Ronald M. Mottl, Democrat of Ohio, used the occasion to challenge FDA Commissioner Arthur Hull Hayes on the delayed promulgation of the recall requirements and quality control regulations called for by the 1980 statute.[30] Both were under consideration by the agency, but Gore and Mottl suggested that Reagan administration devotion to cost-benefit analysis had delayed them unduly. The Wyeth recall and the political pressure generated by congressional attention doubtless helped prompt administration action. The Department of Health and Human Services released both sets of regulations in final form the month after the hearing.[31]

Beneficial but Risky

A central premise of most product regulation is that risks must be balanced against benefits.[32] The FDA's regulation of drugs follows this same reasoning (though the Delaney clause on food additives explicitly staked out a "no risk" position on cancer).[33] All drugs pose some risk of overdose or other improper use, and many can trigger side-effects even when carefully taken. Therefore a major problem is to decide when side-effects are significant enough in quantity and severity to overbalance benefits. Making judgments based on ambiguous evidence is not ideal, and multiple positions can be made to appear reasonable, depending on the relative weights assigned to different factors. A drug may also cause side-effects so rarely that they are hard to identify during clinical trials. Postmarketing surveillance is highly imperfect; the FDA may fail to register and react to side-effects that are rare, mild, or mishandled within the reporting system. And while companies always try to cut their losses by abandoning a dangerously adulterated product, they routinely promote those exhibiting both benefits and dangers.

Visible victims may simplify matters. For some acutely hazardous products, the ratio of obvious harm to benefits is so unfavorable that withdrawal elicits little controversy and may not be particularly hard to implement. Critics will often ask how these products reached consumers in the first place.

In one famous instance, the federal government was primarily responsible. In 1976 not many victims of the swine influenza vaccine had to appear before distribution was halted because no flu epidemic had occurred. By the fall of that year, in the wake of a $135 million national immunization effort, only one new case had shown up that was not directly traceable to contact with pigs.[34] Swine influenza shots commenced in early October.[35] On October 11, "three persons over 70, all with cardiac conditions" died shortly after getting their shots at the same Pittsburgh clinic. A wire service picked up the story, and Allegheny County promptly suspended flu shots, with nine states (though not Pennsylvania) following suit. The panic subsided (with Allegheny County and all nine states relenting) after October 14, when President Ford and his family got televised flu shots. The Pittsburgh deaths were generally attributed to coincidence.

But in late November a Minnesota physician reported a case of a rare ascending paralysis, Guillain-Barré syndrome, following a flu shot. Within a week came three more cases in Minnesota, one fatal. These reports reached the CDC simultaneously with three from Alabama. The following day brought a New Jersey case. The CDC surveillance physician who had received the original call from Minnesota had been unimpressed; by now, though, the agency was paying close attention. On December 16, with the swine flu epidemic still nowhere in sight, the assistant secretary for health suspended the immunization program. Though it likely would have protected most recipients had an epidemic arrived, the vaccine became emblematic of government incompetence. Because the entire supply of vaccine lay in the possession of the manufacturer, government officials, and health professionals (instead of in countless retail stores and home medicine cabinets), withdrawal took place without notable incident.

Withdrawal of beneficial but risky products is common. In the 1980s, for example, the harm done by the nonsteroidal anti-inflammatory drugs Oraflex and Zomax led to withdrawals and provoked congressional criticism of the FDA's drug approval process.[36] In both cases, the manufacturers acted after evidence of adverse reactions and looming publicity made continued marketing infeasible.

Strong support for a product, whether by manufacturers or by consumers, complicates the issue. A constituency of beneficiaries might mobilize to keep a product available. The unproven cancer therapy Laetrile falls into this category, as do some unapproved AIDS drugs; desperate patients can create a formidable constituency even when positive research findings are lacking. Though government-sanctioned, silicone breast implants presented such a situation. In 1991–92 a long-simmering debate over their safety boiled over. The FDA could not move aggressively and swiftly to remove all implants from the market, partly because of uncertainty about the risks associated with the device and partly because of resistance by manufacturers, physicians, and women who argued vehemently for continued availability.[37] Women in Congress, including breast cancer survivors, found themselves in the difficult position of having to "be careful not to argue too hard for availability, which might indicate a lack of safety concerns, or for guarantees of safety, which could make the device virtually unavailable."[38] In April 1992 FDA Commissioner David Kessler steered a middle course, ending a three-month moratorium on the use of silicone implants and allowing continued, but restricted, access to the devices while additional data were collected.[39] The decision would keep implants available for postoperative surgical reconstruction but curtail use for purely cosmetic breast enlargement—a clear attempt to accommodate, in a way justifiable on technical grounds, an unpleasant political tension.

The dietary supplement L-tryptophan was also politically protected. A contaminant in some imported L-tryptophan caused the 1989 outbreak of eosinophilia-myalgia syndrome.[40] State and federal officials acted soon after case reports began arriving.[41] Instances of eosinophilia (an elevated count of white blood cells known as eosinophils) with crippling muscle pain, or myalgia, began to mount beyond the initial three victims after the *Albuquerque Journal* published its first story about the condition on November 7. By November 13 New Mexico officials had banned the supplement, and four days later (in the wake of substantial publicity and pressure from New Mexico Republican senator Pete V. Domenici) the FDA asked for a national recall of all L-tryptophan on the market.[42] On November 11, the FDA had opted for a warning, a move widely criticized as inadequate. But overall the government reacted quickly to an emerging hazard, albeit under pressure, and the overwhelming majority of manufacturers quickly complied.

In the 1970s, as now, L-tryptophan and similar amino acid supplements enjoyed staunch defenders, despite FDA skepticism. In 1970–71 the agency began revising criteria for its so-called GRAS list, which includes a wide variety of commonly used substances that, while not formally approved, are "generally recognized as safe."[43] This list has long included some dietary supplements and at the time included a number of amino acids, L-tryptophan among them. The agency revoked the GRAS status of amino acids in 1972, concluding that "substances intended for human consumption for which limitations are necessary to assure safe use" ought not to make the list.[44]

But L-tryptophan remained available because of agency reversals in court and because Congress intervened to protect supplement manufacturers.[45] In April 1976 Congress amended the Food, Drug, and Cosmetic Act, weakening the FDA's ability to set maximum limits on the potency of vitamins and minerals or to consider them as drugs for regulatory purposes.[46] Senator William Proxmire, Democrat of Wisconsin, championed the changes to block what he derided as "the FDA's and the orthodox nutritionists' efforts to ruin the vitamin industry."[47] Proxmire regarded the recommended daily allowances (RDAs) suggested by the agency, and a move toward more stringent regulation of supplements that exceeded the RDAs by more than 150 percent, as based on inadequate evidence. Congressional supporters could plausibly defend the legislation as proconsumer, a way to maintain easy access to life-enhancing substances in the face of runaway bureaucracy (much as Congress would the following year keep saccharin available by denying the FDA authority to ban it). The FDA was thus understandably reluctant to challenge L-tryptophan aggressively. Had the supplement been more stringently regulated, the 1989 outbreak might have been avoided, either by preventing the specific contamination that triggered it or by discouraging the marketing of L-tryptophan as a nutritional supplement altogether.[48] Subsequent congressional inquiry suggested that over-the-counter bottled L-tryptophan was a de facto drug (with genuine, though not well studied, therapeutic effects) but that no problem of an L-tryptophan deficiency correctable through supplements was known to exist.[49]

The difficulty surrounding withdrawal of the Dalkon Shield may seem strange today. It is now considered the most notorious birth control device ever marketed, evoking much the same horror as the tranquilizer thalidomide. Introduced in 1971 and withdrawn in 1974, the Dalkon Shield produced thousands of damage claims from women alleging that pelvic inflammatory disease brought on by the device caused infertility, spontaneous septic abortion, and other miseries. Eventually, its manufacturer, A. H. Robins, would create a trust fund approaching $2.5 billion to compensate the nearly 200,000 women claiming injury.[50]

But this would happen only after Congress had (encouraged partly by the tragedy) enacted the Medical Device Amendments of 1976, giving the FDA explicit responsibility for premarket approval of the most sensitive and potentially life-threatening devices.[51] The Dalkon Shield entered a market for devices less regulated than that for drugs. Moreover, the company fought to continue sales and deflect blame from its product long after evidence of serious adverse reactions began to accumulate. The company appears to have suppressed and ignored evidence of those reactions. In the face of an advisory committee's reluctance to recommend the strongest possible action against the device in June 1974, the FDA did not request a Class I recall, accepting instead a Robins proposal for a voluntary suspension of sales.[52] In December 1974 company hopes for remarketing the shield appeared to have been vindicated, when the FDA commissioner announced resumed sales under an agreement for more carefully monitored marketing.[53] But in August 1975, citing the marketing hiatus, adverse publicity, and other factors, Robins announced that it was giving up for good on the device.[54]

The L-tryptophan and Dalkon Shield examples point out that the problem of product withdrawal, like any other regulatory action, may be as much political as scientific, because products that harbor dangers may also have advocates. If the perceived benefits of a potentially hazardous product are large enough, explicit advocacy is unnecessary; both common sense and formal analysis counsel that a large-scale permanent withdrawal is unreasonable. The implications of this can be seen most clearly in episodes involving products that have remained widely available despite their hazards. Though one brand of tampon— Rely—was withdrawn during the toxic shock syndrome scare, other brands could and did trigger cases. But no attempt was made to remove all tampons. (For a time, the Rely recall led many to believe, mistakenly, that other brands of tampon posed little or no danger.)[55] Similarly, no one thought to ban aspirin once Reye's syndrome became widely feared, nor did the apparently minute chance of tragic side-effects prompt an outright withdrawal of DPT vaccine. In all three instances, a ban was inappropriate, and debate centered on the problem of public instruction (and, in the case of childhood vaccines, injury compensation and liability protection). Some risks are simply better coped with than eliminated.

Product Approvals

Product approval raises two potentially conflicting desires: to provide careful approval and thus minimize withdrawals while hastening the process when appropriate, as with life-threatening diseases for which existing therapy is inadequate or nonexistent.

Intervening against a damaging product is one thing; reliably preventing such a product from being marketed is another. Given diligent preventive attention by manufacturers, a number of defective products noted above—deficient infant formula, deadly vichyssoise, virulent polio vaccine, tainted L-tryptophan—were doubtless avoidable. The Dalkon Shield tragedy could certainly have been better contained and would never have occurred had the regulatory process for medical devices that exists today been in effect. But, again, questionable products may have defenders, and the very nature of regulation, no matter how stringent, allows officials only to create incentives and checkpoints, not to completely control future behaviors. Moreover, regulatory systems are inevitably better at reaction than anticipation. All such systems have holes, and there is often no way of knowing which will need plugging first, absent a focusing event that clarifies priorities. Even if a potential problem is apparent to some, the incentive to take action may be insufficient unless victimization forces the issue. Over-the-counter Tylenol capsules were long vulnerable to tampering. Even if both the manufacturer and federal regulators had thought of this particular contingency—and it must have occurred to someone at some time or other—the potential problem could reasonably have seemed a far-fetched (or, at least, ever-receding) hypothetical, not worth bothering about in light of competing immediate demands.

The concept of a regulatory system that functions partly by response to unfavorable results, instead of entirely by anticipating them before marketing, doubtless strikes some as messy and unsatisfying, perhaps even immoral. But the size and complexity of the task Congress has given the FDA leaves little practical choice, particularly in an era of tight government budgets. The emphasis on adverse experience reporting shows that such thinking has become accepted doctrine. In a sense, all marketed foods, additives, drugs, and devices enjoy a kind of conditional approval; without apparent victimization, they remain available. Although drugs are subject to a strenuous premarket approval process, including clinical trials, that now averages twelve years, rare side-effects may fail to appear until the product has been licensed.[56] Or side-effects that the agency may have judged acceptable prior to marketing may look different later, as more victims appear and as approval decisions (and any dissent that may have attended them) are cast in a harsh light by congressional overseers and consumer advocates.

Although the importance of postmarketing surveillance and the need to make policy partly in response to evidence of harm have been acknowledged, the FDA's political environment has inclined the agency mostly toward avoiding approval of harmful substances. Not that the agency simply waits for bad things to happen and then reacts. Because the agency has been so cautious in approvals, some critics complain it has damaged public health by keeping beneficial substances off the market longer than necessary.[57] Occasional academic and industry critics of "drug lag" have been visible and vocal as far back as the 1970s.[58] But for years their voices were largely drowned out by the consumer movement and its allies in Congress, insistent upon caution. In hearing after hearing, year after year, Congress told the FDA mostly one thing: Do not approve, or allow to remain accessible, products—whether foods, food additives, drugs, or medical devices—that cause demonstrable harm to identifiable individuals. Each instance of visible, and thus media-worthy, harm allowed the prostringency coalition to reiterate this message.

Beginning in 1981, two forces appeared that would challenge the existing orientation dramatically. One was the Reagan administration, which was determined to turn back what it viewed as a tide of costly overregulation that had swelled during the 1960s and 1970s. Through appointments, budget and personnel cuts, statutory interpretation, and vastly enhanced White House and OMB review of proposed rules, the administration conducted an unprecedented frontal assault on the regulatory status quo.[59]

The second force was the AIDS calamity. By the mid-1980s the epidemic was claiming thousands of new victims each year with no end in sight. Far more than other diseases, AIDS gave rise to a vigorous, even militant, movement composed of people with AIDS, their friends, and loved ones. Urban communities of gay men, hit particularly hard by the epidemic and already both self-aware and somewhat alienated from the larger society, perceived the government's response as dreadfully inadequate. As the White House eschewed formal recognition of AIDS as a major health threat in the early years, with President Reagan refusing even to mention the epidemic in public, AIDS activists found allies in Congress and among health professionals. These activists, in concert with government deregulation advocates, succeeded in legitimizing an alternative to the dogma of extreme caution for drug approvals—at least for AIDS. In the latter years of his chairmanship of the House Government Operations Subcommittee on Human Resources and Intergovernmental Relations, Ted Weiss, a key member of the coalition otherwise demanding regulatory stringency from the FDA, supported making AIDS drugs available more quickly to those who needed them—perhaps not a surprising development given the gay presence in Weiss's Manhattan district.[60] Even Sidney Wolfe of the Public Citizen Health Research Group, a consistent Weiss ally, would petition the agency in 1990 to expedite its review of ddI and ddC, two then-experimental AIDS drugs.[61]

The regulatory process that leads to a drug's distribution can be hastened in two ways. One is to contract the time, or number of steps, necessary for review, perhaps making available extraordinary resources on an ad hoc basis. The government and Burroughs Wellcome did just that to get AZT into trials and to speed up distribution once effectiveness against HIV appeared to have been established. The other way is to circumvent review, at least partially, by making drugs available before or during regulatory scrutiny. Both approaches became FDA policy largely because of AIDS.[62] The obvious constraint on both approaches, and on any review process, is that substances must exist before they can be reviewed. And only about 20 percent of all drugs put into phase 1 tests for toxicity survive through the more elaborate phase 2 and phase 3 tests for safety and efficacy and thus complete the review process.

In the late 1980s a combination of government officials, disease advocates, and supporters of regulatory relief propelled important reforms in response to AIDS. One was expedited review, under a more flexible risk-benefit framework, of medications for life-threatening or severely debilitating illnesses. After Burroughs Wellcome approached the FDA about interest in developing an anti-HIV product in early 1985, the agency began to communicate closely with and to assist drug developers, though some benefited far more than others.[63] In September 1986 the FDA established a special 1-AA classification to give AIDS drugs top priority in the review process.[64] Sensitive both to business concerns and the plight of the desperately ill, the president's Task Force on Regulatory Relief, chaired by Vice President George Bush, in August 1988 requested the FDA to formalize a policy for "expediting the marketing of new therapies intended to treat AIDS and other life-threatening illnesses."[65] The agency published an interim rule the following October, and expedited review became agency policy. The FDA was to make itself as helpful as possible to drug sponsors early in the development and evaluation process and to consider "the severity of the disease and the absence of satisfactory alternative therapy" when deciding on approval.[66]

A second change was the so-called treatment IND, through which an Investigational New Drug (one still undergoing preapproval clinical study) could reach limited populations. Unlike expedited review, the treatment IND was conceived as a bridge to final approval that allowed early access to promising therapies before all the data were in, a power the FDA had informally exercised earlier. Even before an agency rule took effect in June 1987, about four thousand patients had received AZT in this manner.[67] The advent of the treatment IND rule did not presage a flood of new drugs. As one congressional committee later complained, during the year after the regulation, only one drug (trimetrexate, for AIDS-related pneumonia) received treatment IND status. Since then, few other AIDS drugs that later won full approval successfully crossed the treatment IND bridge.

A third reform, the so-called parallel track concept, originated in the AIDS activist community and received a sudden surprise endorsement by National Institute of Allergy and Infectious Diseases (NIAID) Director Anthony S. Fauci in June 1989. Formally announced in May 1990, it aimed to make promising new AIDS drugs available "through studies without concurrent control groups to monitor drug safety that are conducted in parallel with the principal controlled clinical investigations." It promised expanded availability even "when the evidence for effectiveness is less than that generally required for a treatment IND."[68] A major concern was to craft the policy so that the availability of drugs outside of clinical trials did not rob drug sponsors of their ability to recruit trial participants. In October 1992 the FDA approved the antiretroviral drug d4T (stavudine) to be the first available under parallel track.[69] (The drug's final approval came in June 1994).[70]

In June 1989 the FDA for the first time based approval of a drug—aerosolized pentamidine, to prevent pneumonia—entirely on data from community-based research.[71] The following September the secretary of health and human services announced the early release of ddI, an antiretroviral drug that showed signs of helping patients for whom AZT was not an option. That occurred after negotiations among the sponsor (Bristol-Meyers), the FDA, and AIDS activists.[72] Activists also pushed for full FDA licensing of both ddI and ddC even though (and to some extent, precisely because) clinical trials had been slow to proceed.[73] In short, the AIDS constituency extracted meaningful flexibility from regulators.

Unfortunately, structural and procedural innovation, no matter how well intended or how grounded in thoughtful prospective analysis, can almost never guarantee substantive progress. Outcomes have proved ambiguous. By 1991, ten years after formal recognition of the epidemic, the FDA had approved nine imperfect or limited AIDS-related drugs. By spring 1994 the AIDS Clinical Trials Information Service listed twenty-one FDA-approved AIDS drugs. Two—Bactrim/Septra and pyrimethamine—had been relabeled for use in persons with HIV because diseases for which they had been approved happened also to be opportunistic infections. Pentamidine had been used to combat the occasional case of *Pneumocystis* pneumonia well before the HIV epidemic. AZT, the first approved drug to attack the HIV virus itself, proved a major disappointment. Many people with AIDS either could not tolerate it or developed AZT-resistant strains of HIV, generating understandable demands for more therapeutic options, which the availability of ddI and ddC did little to quell. Many activists also saw the treatment IND as little more than FDA public relations.[74]

Some observers worry that the effort to make AIDS drugs available quickly could unduly compromise safety and efficacy.[75] With a life-threatening terror such as AIDS, risk-benefit inquiry acquires a complexity absent for most drugs. Not everything claiming to benefit anyone terminally ill can be released. To do so may give the unscrupulous a strong incentive to exploit desperate patients. But excessively quick approvals remain hypothetical, and both the practicalities and politics of the approval process suggest that this will continue to hold for some time to come. The practical problem is that AIDS-related drugs have been trickling slowly out of the laboratory and through clinical trials. Politically, these drugs have displayed various risks and limitations, but organized people with AIDS have concentrated on multiplying their therapeutic options, not on policing them. And most other drug approvals remain embedded in the same politics of stringency that produced complaints of drug lag in the first place. Despite tantalizing indications that disease constituencies outside the gay community might start to "act up," few had.[76] However, the FDA realized that, given increased resources, review times for many drugs could be significantly shortened, something that regulators, business, and patients clearly wanted.

Process Regulation

Regulation that challenges the established practices of an entire industry or profession, perhaps threatening it with unaccustomed inconvenience or increased costs, proves especially difficult.[77] Other things being equal, the larger the number of policy targets, the more elusive will be policy consensus. And the incentive for organized dissent or resistance among regulated interests increases with the perceived stakes of each participant and the sense that collective action could successfully defend them. Regulated interests are often politically entrenched well in advance of any specific proposal and can therefore influence both particular regulations and the agenda-setting process that generates them. For many activities, particularly where the public remains ignorant and opposition unmobilized, virtual self-regulation is the norm.[78]

Such factors have been apparent on two related fronts of the battle against AIDS. One is the effort to guard supplies of blood and blood products against HIV contamination. The other is the attempt to protect workers against HIV infection contracted on the job.

The Safety of Supplies

One of the more tragic responses to the emerging epidemic came from within the blood products industry during the early 1980s. In the year after the epidemic had been formally recognized, AIDS cases seemed to be clustered among homosexual and bisexual men, injecting drug users, and Haitians. By the summer of 1982, however, the CDC was aware of another category—hemophiliacs, persons with a chronic and moderate-to-severe disorder of the blood-clotting mechanism. In July 1982 the CDC published accounts of three cases of *Pneumocystis* pneumonia among hemophiliacs, noting that this ailment "has not been previously reported among hemophilia patients who have had no other underlying diseases and have not had therapy commonly associated with immunosuppression."[79] The following December saw reports of four more hemophiliac AIDS cases, all of whom had received clotting factor concentrates to help control their conditions.[80] The same month the CDC noted a case of "possible transfusion-associated" AIDS in a twenty-month-old infant who developed "unexplained cellular immunodeficiency and opportunistic infection" after multiple transfusions, including platelets derived from the blood of someone who subsequently developed AIDS.[81] The infant's parents were "heterosexual non-Haitians" without a history of intravenous drug abuse. Both parents, and a sibling, were in good health, and there had been no known contact with an AIDS patient.

Although the specific pathogen that causes AIDS would not be identified until early 1984, federal officials and the blood products industry confronted the probability that the disease was blood-borne much earlier. Action to safeguard blood and blood products emerged hesitantly, accompanied by considerable denial of the problem's potential severity and a strong inclination toward voluntary action rather than stringent regulation. By mid-1988 approximately twenty-four hundred known persons with symptomatic AIDS (and a far larger number of persons with HIV) had contracted it through exposure to blood and its various derivatives.[82] The presidential commission charged with studying the epidemic concluded that "the initial response of the nation's blood banking industry to the possibility of contamination of the nation's blood by a new infectious agent was unnecessarily slow."[83]

Beyond any doubt, those most harmed were hemophiliacs. A single dose of clotting factor may derive from the pooled plasma of thousands of donors. Severe hemophilia may, in turn, require dozens of doses of clotting factor in a year, thus exposing a patient to the blood of tens of thousands of donors. Such figures led in an obvious and tragic direction. In 1990 congressional testimony, the executive director of the

National Hemophilia Foundation reported that half of all hemophiliacs had contracted HIV and that 70–80 percent of persons with severe hemophilia had.[84]

In the early 1980s some blood industry representatives were reluctant to acknowledge, at least publicly, the potential scope of the problem.[85] During a blood industry meeting at the CDC in January 1983, the head of the New York Blood Center chastised other participants: "Don't overstate the facts. There are, at most, three cases of AIDS from blood donations, and the evidence in two of those cases is very soft. And there are only a handful of cases among hemophiliacs."[86] Later that month, the three major blood collecting organizations issued a joint statement that said, "Fewer than 10 cases of AIDS with possible linkage to transfusion have been seen despite approximately 10 million transfusions per year," implying that transfusion recipients only had a one-in-a-million risk of getting AIDS.[87] (In 1985, after an HIV blood test had become available, one of the organizations, the American Red Cross, would survey donations at nine of its regional centers and determine prevalence of HIV infection to be about 380 per million.)[88]

In the years before a direct HIV antibody test became available, most of the industry was disinclined to use an existing surrogate test capable of detecting abnormal ratios of T cells (a kind of white blood cell important to the immune response), a phenomenon common in the blood of persons who later developed AIDS. The Stanford University Blood Bank became the first in the nation to adopt this test in July 1983. The test's usefulness and resistance to it by much of the blood industry were recounted by Dr. Edgar G. Engleman, medical director of the Stanford blood bank, in congressional testimony several years later:

[We knew that our testing] . . . would probably not detect 100 percent of AIDS carriers and would identify some individuals who were not carriers at all, [but] we nonetheless felt that the benefits of preventing at least some AIDS-contaminated blood from entering the blood supply outweighed the fact that a small amount of normal blood was unavoidably discarded and that each unit of blood cost $6 more. In our view the blood banking community failed to recognize that we could not afford to wait until the causative agent was discovered or until the perfect test was developed. . . . In an attempt to publicly bring the matter out for discussion in the blood banking community, in the summer of 1983 we submitted an abstract on the subject for presentation to the annual national meeting of the American Association of Blood Banks (AABB). . . . Although we were disappointed that our abstract was rejected for presentation at the meeting, it was particularly distressing to discover later that the subject of transfusion-associated AIDS wasn't even on the meeting's program. . . .

The efficacy of our screening program . . . [was] demonstrated in the summer of 1983. Follow-up interviews revealed that several donors whose blood was excluded from transfusion on the basis of our screening test had, in fact, donated despite belonging to AIDS high-risk groups. The point was further underscored in early 1984 when we learned that a donor whose blood our test had rejected had been hospitalized with AIDS some 8 months after his attempted blood donation. . . . We retrospectively tested frozen blood from donors whose T cell tests had been abnormal, and found that the T cell test had successfully identified approximately two-thirds of the HIV infected individuals who had donated blood—not a perfect result, but significantly better than doing no testing at all.[89]

In March 1983 the FDA announced new recommendations to reduce the risk of transmitting AIDS through transfusions. The agency urged the issuance of a pamphlet to donors giving information on risk factors, symptoms, and means of dissemination. The donor could then decide if he or she were at high risk and refrain from donating. Two years later, when the HIV antibody test became available, the FDA recommended its use by blood collection facilities, but a regulation did not become final until January 1988.[90] In the interim, as one critical account later noted, "some blood banks delayed using it and others did not test thousands of pints of blood already in their inventories."[91]

Hesitancy by the blood services industry reflected caution on the part of organizations with significant stakes to protect. Distinctions between different segments of the industry must be made. The "source plasma" sector, which is commercial, consists mainly of facilities that collect plasma (more formally known as plasmapheresis centers) and fractionators, who separate it into a number of different products, including clotting factor.[92] Economist Ross D. Eckert argued that the plasma sector was notably more inclined to embrace tough screening standards for high-risk donors than the whole blood and components sector, served mainly by volunteer donors.[93] This seems to reflect partly the plasma sector's early recognition of the far greater risk-per-dose inherent in its products and partly that sector's confidence that paid donors could be found even if some high-risk persons had to be turned away. The whole blood sector, meanwhile, was anxious about maintaining access to its voluntary contributors. The fear of driving away donors and of rejecting too much usable blood through inaccurate testing was an ongoing concern of the blood service industry throughout the debates of the early and mid-1980s on safeguarding supplies.

But in the face of a public health emergency, how did the industry manage to continue operating as it wished? Eckert pointed to an answer in the routine politics of blood services regulation. The FDA is not a captive of regulated interests, but they have been hugely influential, particularly to the extent that others, such as consumers, remain largely unorganized and inattentive. As late as 1989 the eleven voting members of the FDA's blood products advisory committee included, in the words of one member, "a hematologist, a pathologist, an economist, five medical school faculty in various specialties, and three blood bankers, one of whom was chairman. . . . The committee's 'camp followers' consist mainly of blood bankers and the representatives of their three trade associations, manufacturers and the representative of their trade association, journalists, and financial people. Representatives of consumers who are heavy users of blood and blood products appear before us only occasionally."[94] Not surprisingly, the advice emanating from the committee reflected strong sensitivity to the concerns of blood banks. One result of the restraint inherent in this system was a further dissemination of HIV-tainted blood to an extent incalculable but surely not trivial. By the time retired tennis star Arthur Ashe acknowledged his own transfusion-linked HIV infection, in April 1992, the number of blood products-associated AIDS cases stood at about forty-eight hundred.[95] Much testing that should have been done was delayed, and some donors who should have been notified quickly and carefully of their infections were not.

In later years these early failings were largely though imperfectly corrected. Screening for HIV is now mandatory and had been widely adopted even before it was. The risk of receiving HIV from blood that has been properly screened is not zero but low, perhaps 1 in 40,000 transfused units according to a 1988 estimate by the CDC.[96] In mid-1990 CDC Director William Roper noted that "investigation of AIDS cases who received blood transfusions after screening began in March

1985 has identified only 11 who were infected from these transfusions."[97] Clotting factors were also made safer through processing to kill HIV.[98] Some hazard remains, however. Blood banks continue to commit errors.[99] Some persons at risk for HIV infection continue to donate blood despite attempts to fend them off with both education and questioning at time of donation. And the test is vulnerable to false negatives among newly infected persons who have not yet developed the antibodies to which the tests react.[100] Estimates of full-blown AIDS cases that stem from post-1985 blood donations do not account for a much larger unknown number of HIV infections that have resulted.[101]

The Health of Workers

The issue of occupational exposure to HIV proved even more politically complex because of a proliferation of contending voices, each with its own priorities and fears. Occupational safety and health regulation has long been an area of keen political competition, chiefly between organized labor, which is the primary political constituency of the Occupational Safety and Health Administration (OSHA), and business lobbies, which were anxious to constrain the costs regulation might impose on their members.[102] Any proposed rule was certain to spur interest among a wide variety of affected parties, including labor, management, and assorted professions. The rulemaking would have to take account of everyone who might be exposed to infected blood: physicians, dentists, nurses, prison guards, laboratory technicians, firemen, police, blood bank staff, mortuary personnel, and others. And a rule of such scope, with any real teeth, was bound to strike some as "excessively rigid and burdensome," the language the AABB used during congressional testimony to describe the proposal.[103] The multiplicity of settings and circumstances in which someone might be exposed to the major pathogens of concern, HIV and hepatitis B virus (HBV), guaranteed not only that the proceedings would be lengthy and complex, but also that interest groups would offer competing views on the degree of regulatory stringency warranted.

The blood-borne pathogen proposal, OSHA's first foray into the regulation of biological hazards, combined three protective strategies: (1) engineering controls that "isolate or remove the hazard from the workplace,"[104] (2) work practice controls to "reduce the likelihood of exposure by altering the manner in which a task is performed,"[105] and (3) the use of personal protective equipment or clothing worn by employees. Historically, both OSHA's industrial hygienists and the agency's union clientele have strongly preferred the first strategy to the others, and particularly to the third.[106] But many companies and some economists have viewed personal protection as both effective and much less costly than engineering controls. The reliance on multiple strategies sprang from the technical and political complexity that underlay the agency's effort; given the virtually endless number of specific work settings and situations the standard would have to address, all three seemed useful. The writing of individual rules by OSHA has always been far more contentious for health than for safety, and relatively few health-focused rules have survived the cauldron of competing demands.

The rulemaking process began in earnest in September 1986, when several unions, including the American Federation of State, County, and Municipal Employees (AFSCME), petitioned OSHA to protect workers against exposure to infectious disease. AFSCME was motivated by reported instances of worker exposure to potentially hazardous blood and by the apparently uneven application of the CDC's guidelines for protecting workers against such exposure.[107] The CDC could recommend precautions, but only OSHA could require them. Labor deemed inadequate a 1983 set of voluntary OSHA guidelines for employers, intended to deal with HBV exposure.

A long period of political haggling preceded the May 1989 announcement of a proposed rule. Concerned about HBV exposure, the 1986 union petitions called for an emergency temporary standard (ETS) requiring employers to provide to employees, free of charge, an expensive immunization series. OSHA denied the petitions but promised to pursue a formal rulemaking.[108] In early 1988, after four months of negotiation, the Office of Management and Budget denied OSHA's request to conduct its own infection control survey.[109] Congressional Democrats chairing subcommittees with oversight jurisdiction over OSHA blamed OMB for delaying and weakening the agency's proposal, unnecessarily jeopardizing lives in a misguided obsession with costs.[110]

The May 1989 announcement triggered a new round of objections. The organized physicians, dentists, blood banks, and hospitals tended to emphasize the proposal's potential costs and stringency; they found it wanting while applauding its intent. The American Dental Association argued that "the dental profession is at very low risk of contracting infectious bloodborne diseases."[111] The blood products industry was inclined to see its donor population as harboring no greater risk than the population at large, with the blood of frequent donors being safer than average in light of the regular monitoring such donors would undergo.[112] Unions and other associations representing health care employees were more supportive, particularly of engineering controls to minimize accidental needle punctures and other sharp object injuries. The AFSCME health and safety coordinator accused the agency of an effort to deemphasize such controls, citing as evidence explicit language indicating a preference for them that had appeared in a preannouncement draft of the proposed rule but was later dropped.[113] A pervasive complication in the deliberations was the unavoidable need to address, both rhetorically and substantively, events that were unlikely or of uncertain probability. Although both corrections officers and mental health personnel could conceivably contract HIV from a bite by an agitated inmate, no confirmed instance of such an event was known. (Bites had been known to transmit HBV.) Similarly, infection could theoretically result from exposure to blood aerosols, though the probability was widely regarded to be low—immeasurably low. Even real events, such as confirmed HIV infection from needle injuries, had tended to be so scarce and scary as to shed more heat than light on actual risk levels.

In December 1991, acting under the pressure of a formal statutory deadline imposed by congressional appropriators the previous year, OSHA promulgated its final rule on occupational exposures to bloodborne pathogens.[114] Relying on all three control strategies, the rule endorsed the principle of "universal precautions" in which "all human blood and certain human body fluids are treated as if known to be infectious for HIV, HBV, and other bloodborne pathogens."[115] It also required that employers make vaccine and medical follow-up available at no charge to any employee who has "occupational exposure" (meaning "reasonably anticipated" contact) with HBV.[116] These two infection control strategies, universal precautions and vaccination, had earlier been judged effective in lowering the risk of hepatitis transmission in health care settings.[117]

Conclusion

When the target is a single product line or batch, the manufacturer has an incentive to make changes, and governmental action is technically feasible, regulatory objectives such as product withdrawal are likely to be achievable quickly, with little resistance. For more complex hazards, however, the mechanics and politics of regulation become far more cumbersome. When self-interested parties with power over the regulatory process perceive specific strategies of hazard abatement as inconvenient or threatening, they will resist those strategies. And such resistance impedes the ability of government to act quickly.

Three kinds of regulatory situations are more vexing than relatively simple bad batch problems. One involves a product that, whatever its dangers, yields benefits as well, at least for some well-defined and organizable constituency.[118] Aspirin was not a reasonable candidate for withdrawal in the 1980s, despite its highly publicized association with Reye's syndrome. Nor did it make sense to remove tampons in the wake of the toxic shock syndrome panic. DPT vaccine causes harm only rarely at most (though as the advocacy group Dissatisfied Parents Together points out at the top of every newsletter: "When it happens to *your* child, the risks are 100%").[119] The vaccine's offsetting benefits were clear to a broad spectrum of health professionals and to the general public. Had the FDA made silicone breast implants completely unavailable, the agency would probably have found its position politically untenable.

A second challenge is hastened product approval. The HIV epidemic made faster approvals a cause that proregulation liberals were inclined to support, transforming the politics of drug regulation.[120] AIDS prodded government officials to do something that, despite repeated complaints and multiple studies, had never before been given such urgency: to think hard about ways to speed regulatory review of new drugs. Experience accumulated in hastening AIDS drugs ultimately helped to convince the FDA leadership that, given access to enhanced resources, similar efficiencies might be achieved more broadly.[121] (A direct result was the Prescription Drug User Fee Act of 1992, under which pharmaceutical manufacturers would be assessed fees for the review of drugs, with the funds raised to be plowed back into the agency's coffers to hire the personnel—an additional six hundred employees, according to supporters—needed to expedite reviews.[122] It was anticipated that review times could be reduced from twenty to twelve months, with scrutiny of so-called breakthrough drugs completed in as little as six months.[123] But even this pathblazing legislation could do nothing directly to address the problem of getting new drugs developed and submitted to the FDA in the first place.)

A third difficult situation requires broad (perhaps industry-wide or multi-industry) process quality reform. A plethora of participants offering competing claims about the kind and degree of regulatory change appropriate sets the stage for sluggish policymaking. This marks a vast and telling difference between the bad blood episodes and the virtually instant and universal embrace of major reform elicited by the Tylenol poisonings.

Seven

Research

FOR PRACTICAL and institutional reasons, biomedical research remains an awkward and uncertain response to hazards of every sort. Private sector drug sponsors and university-based researchers may face incentives to avoid certain kinds of research or to conduct it in ways that frustrate laymen. A more significant constraint is that preventive and ameliorative technologies are inherently elusive even when controversy is absent, commitment unwavering, and research techniques creative. The inputs that can be manipulated—funding, procedures, priorities, leadership—cannot guarantee desirable technology. At the heart of research lies search, not production.

Nevertheless, serious and persistent threats to public health are likely to spur some sustained government-sponsored scientific inquiry, and emergent public health hazards are no exception. But unduly hazardous consumer products are far less likely than infectious diseases to prompt such research. One reason is that a health problem may exist only for discrete units or batches of the product. In that event, withdrawal suffices. And those kinds of hazards may be technically straightforward, like the equipment defect that punctured cans of Alaska salmon in 1980 and allowed deadly botulinum toxin to develop. (A Belgian man died after eating it.)[1] A second reason is that even when the precise cause of a product's adverse effects is not evident, the appropriate response is usually to abandon the product and allow the private sector to look for less hazardous alternatives. Asking government scientists and peer review panelists to direct significant resources toward analyzing why a particular drug induced unacceptable adverse reactions usually makes little sense. The ready availability of substitute therapies particularly undermines the rationale for government to make the perfection of any given drug or device a priority.

Some products are not so easily dismissed. When product withdrawal is unreasonable, sustained government involvement becomes more defensible. Reye's syndrome, toxic shock syndrome, and vaccine injuries necessitated ongoing consumer education; they also justified government-funded research. Novel infectious diseases are similar. Legionnaires' disease, chronic fatigue syndrome, and Lyme disease have all drawn government research support—the latter two largely through lobbying by grassroots organizations of affected persons.[2] And by the late 1980s funding for AIDS research had grown into a major focus of the NIH budget. For AIDS and other diseases, however, the paucity of tangible benefits has proved frustrating.

Funding

In recent decades, the federal commitment to biomedical research has mushroomed, although budget constraints and increasing costs took a particular toll after 1980. In fiscal year 1993 the National Institutes of Health budget stood at more than $10.3 billion, up from $4.3 billion in 1983. But there occurred only modest real dollar growth in the NIH budget during the 1980s, and much of that reflected an exploding federal commitment to AIDS research.[3]

Federal funding for science of all kinds is unavoidably political in multiple senses of the word, even when expert peer review is both well established and consistently applied, partly because public money is being dispensed in response to concerted advocacy by organized claimants. Funding, moreover, requires refined judgment about how to balance competing needs and values given the available resources. And the many different players in the funding game—Congress, the NIH, the recipient individuals and institutions—may incur credit or blame and may prosper or decline as a direct result of the patterns and levels of funding and their outcomes. Thus politics is inherent in science funding even when Congress is not investigating fraud and waste, earmarking money for pet projects, or responding to orchestrated lobbying.[4]

Scientific research relevant to emergent health hazards occurs in various locales and is not solely an NIH activity. CDC laboratories have, for example, played important roles in the fight against AIDS, Lyme disease, and Legionnaires' disease. Private sector biomedical research is also a vast and rapidly growing enterprise. In recent years the NIH has provided about one-third of national spending on health research and development, while private industry has grown to about one-half.[5]

Extramural funding from the NIH reaches researchers through three vehicles: grants, contracts, and cooperative agreements.[6] In agency parlance, grant applications and contract proposals are mutually distinct, and individual institutes solicit them through requests for applications (RFAs) or requests for proposals (RFPs) published in the weekly *NIH Guide for Grants and Contracts*. The NIH also sustains outside scientists through its Division of Research Grants, primarily responsible for reviewing the many unsolicited (that is, investigator-initiated) applications that arrive. In fiscal year 1992 the NIH spent about $6.2 billion in research and development grants and $805 million in contracts.[7] All extramural applications are subject to the same basic review process. An initial review committee composed of nongovernment scientists evaluates and scores applications, in effect making the primary recommendation about projects to receive support. Only after an advisory committee ratifies (and perhaps adjusts) these recommendations do funds flow to investigators.[8]

An emergent health hazard can sorely try such a system. Until AIDS, few had demanded quick technological benefits from the NIH, not even during the so-called War on Cancer in the early 1970s.[9] Fast response was the purview of the CDC and the FDA. The NIH is a decentralized basic research institution whose working priorities emerge largely from the external scientists who apply for funds and sit on review committees; suddenly prominent health hazards have typically been of only tenuous relevance to the NIH mission.

A new or newly prominent hazard that might spread quickly suggests a need for fast adjustment in operating priorities. The NIH can reshape its funding in three principal and complementary ways to address a problem. It embraced all three—higher, faster, and more coordinated funding—in response to the HIV epidemic. Why and how it did this, and with what results, is instructive. Under significant external pressure, the agency pursued significant reform in both processes and priorities.

Like the FDA in regulatory approvals, the NIH embraced a fast-track approach for AIDS research funding, which it viewed as a concrete and feasible response consistent with both a novel situation and the agency's mission. The political trick was to hasten funding in a way that would not harm the agency, alienate scientists, or provoke avoidable controversy.

Predictably, the agency's initial response was hesitant and incremental. Fairly soon after the epidemic was recognized, the NIH began turning some of its own resources toward research into the new and interesting syndrome later labeled AIDS, reassigning intramural scientists who had been funded to perform other work.[10] As it became clear that the disease was likely viral, NIH researchers were intrigued. The laboratory of tumor cell biology led by Robert Gallo of the National Cancer Institute began work in the spring of 1982, operating under the suspicion that a retrovirus might be the culprit.[11] The NCI also started giving small awards to study AIDS to outside scientists in September 1982, when it announced eleven such grants.[12] The first important extramural effort by the National Institute of Allergy and Infectious Diseases (NIAID) was to announce a request for proposals in May 1983 for the Multicenter AIDS Cohort Studies (MACS). These contracts, awarded relatively quickly in September 1983, went "to five locations around the country to follow cohorts of homosexual men and to examine the natural history and epidemiology of the disease."[13] The NIAID's first RFP offering support to AIDS treatment evaluation units (subsequently known as AIDS clinical trials groups) was not announced until the fall of 1985, with contracts awarded in June 1986. Congressional critics and AIDS activists would judge these efforts inadequate.[14]

The NIH made a modest effort at speeding up the selection of funding recipients in the early 1980s, using mail balloting to avoid the delay of convening busy scientists for review meetings.[15] As the epidemic grew, so did demands for saving time. During its 1985 congressional reauthorization, for example, the NIH was strongly encouraged to process research support more quickly.[16] The Presidential Commission on the Human Immunodeficiency Virus Epidemic delivered the same message in 1988.[17] The agency's position was difficult. Some researchers, fearful that their applications might receive incomplete consideration, wanted to avoid any expedited process for their submissions.[18]

As Congress approached the enactment of major AIDS amendments in the Health Omnibus Programs Extension of 1988, NIH officials insisted that any required speed-up be realistic. On average, thirteen months would elapse between the publication of an RFA and a funding decision, and the Senate Labor and Human Resources staff initially wanted this time cut in half. The 1988 law would require that AIDS-targeted research funds be awarded not later than six months after the close of the three-month solicitation period. Once an RFA or RFP was announced, the agency would have up to nine months to make its awards.

This reform, aptly called ASAP (for Accelerated Solicitation to Award Program), proved a feasible, albeit very limited, help in the search for usable knowledge. Through ASAP, the NIH could reliably dictate, monitor, and coordinate a set of prescribed activities toward a definite and well-understood end: a funding decision by a certain time. The NIH could assure that, with rare exceptions, the nine-month deadline would work, and without compromising the time available for scientific scrutiny.[19] Simple administrative shortcuts helped. Additional executive secretaries (the NIH staff scientists who manage review committees) can be assigned to conduct ad hoc review meetings if necessary to meet the ASAP deadline. If applications are numerous, or particularly complex, two executive secretaries can be assigned the tasks ordinarily performed by one. The NIH got OMB approval to request multiple copies of AIDS-related applications to save several days otherwise necessary for copying and routing documents. The thrice yearly receipt dates for the unsolicited AIDS applications reviewed by study sections under the Division of Research Grants were set at January 2, May 1, and September 1, each a full month before others are due, allowing the recording and assignment units in the agency to be used for AIDS while administrative capacity is otherwise minimally stressed. The NIAID might also forewarn the scientific community of an impending announcement, giving potential applicants more preparation time. And the NIAID's AIDS Review Committee, but not the study sections, began screening applications early in the peer review process to eliminate those clearly uncompetitive—a process called triage.[20]

ASAP was a direct result of the unique political climate wrought by the HIV epidemic. Organized disease constituencies have traditionally promoted the creation of new institutes and funds, sometimes earmarked for particular ailments such as sickle cell anemia. AIDS generated unprecedented demand for action. But creating a whole new institute would have been problematic on practical grounds (given the existence of the NIAID and the crisis atmosphere) and arguably less effective than a more decentralized approach drawing on the strengths of existing NIH components.[21]

Other emergent health hazards have never come close to rallying this kind of pressure for speedy decisionmaking. The various advocacy constituencies have been smaller, weaker, and much less militant. Despite some media attention, a national perception of crisis has understandably been absent for such problems as Lyme disease, chronic fatigue syndrome, Reye's syndrome, and vaccine injuries. To the chagrin of disease advocates, these problems have not been generally perceived as national crises at all, so a difference of a few months in the funding process would matter little. Moreover, the amounts of money focused on emergent public health hazards other than AIDS have been unexceptional and therefore accommodated within routine NIH funding practices without appreciable stress or controversy. A lag of some years occurs between initial publicity and victimization and extramural funding.[22] Reported cases of Reye's syndrome peaked in 1980 and declined markedly thereafter. Extramural funding for projects wholly or largely concerned with RS went from about $200,000 per fiscal year in the mid-1970s to slightly more than $600,000 in fiscal 1980. Only in fiscal years 1983 and 1984 did funding exceed $2 million, remaining in excess of $1 million annually for the rest of the decade. Extramural funding for toxic shock syndrome research does not appear in NIH data until fiscal year 1985, when two grants totaling $153,631 were funded, fully five years after the 1979–80 tampon scare. And not until fiscal 1989 would an epidemiology and disease control study section support work by Anthony Komaroff of the Brigham and Women's Hospital in Boston concerned with the prevalence of chronic fatigue syndrome.[23]

Too Much Money for AIDS?

During the decade after 1981, the size of the NIH's AIDS budget grew massively. For fiscal year 1982 total AIDS-related spending was $3.3 million. As the epidemic spread, attracted more press coverage, and generated more effective lobbying, this commitment ballooned by fiscal year 1991 to more than $800 million.[24] The unprecedented rapidity and scale of the increases, undertaken in the face of persistently severe fiscal constraint, prompted claims that AIDS research had begun to swallow too large a slice of the funding pie.[25]

This complaint mainly rests on five observations. First, the overwhelming majority of people with AIDS in the United States have been concentrated among identifiably narrow social strata—male homosexuals, injecting drug users, and hemophiliacs (along with the offspring and sexual partners of these groups). Second, because HIV is not transmitted via casual contact and the vast majority of Americans do not fall into these groups, they face an extremely small risk of HIV infection now that blood donations are regularly tested for antibodies to the virus. According to one study published exactly a decade after the epidemic was recognized, the rate of new infections may have declined markedly beginning in the mid-1980s.[26] Third, while the epidemic received uneven official attention, especially during the first years after its discovery, a vigorous and demonstrably effective lobbying network developed. Fourth, some other public health problems (for example, cancer, heart disease, hypertension, accidents) yield higher annual mortality, morbidity, and social cost than does AIDS. Fifth, attention to AIDS has siphoned money away from other problems such as these. As one critic of the high priority accorded AIDS wrote:

> AIDS research has now drained cancer research to a point where the [National Cancer Institute's] ability to fund promising new research proposals is less than at any time in the past two decades. During fiscal year 1989, only 25 percent of cancer grant applications approved by review committees will receive funding. During the 1970s, between 43 percent and 60 percent of such approved grants were funded. Two top NCI doctors left the agency in 1988, partly in frustration over this. "They bled cancer to feed AIDS in terms of people's time," complained one.[27]

These factors are compelling but do not prove that AIDS has received too much. The claim of excessive spending is at least partly embedded in a common cynicism about politics. Activities for which organized lobbying leads to dramatic jumps in funding are suspect. And in politics the emotional content of an issue tends to matter as much as its substance.[28]

Regarding the first few years of the recognized HIV epidemic, both reasonable caution and raw fear argued for a strong, even obsessive, response. Unlike cancer and heart disease, already the focus of major long-standing research commitments supported with public and private funding, AIDS was a new problem. It was both "the first major [new] life-threatening infectious disease epidemic faced by the United States in decades" and "the first such epidemic since the advent of modern biology and the growth of the national biomedical research enterprise."[29] No dedicated research infrastructure existed. Moreover, AIDS was not only newly recognized and infectious but also appeared to be invariably fatal.[30]

An editorial in the *New Republic* argued that, as with many kinds of research, the long-term benefits of AIDS work remain unforeseeable:

> Biomedical research cannot be narrowly compartmentalized; spin-offs frequently develop in areas that seem superficially unrelated. . . . Spending on Richard Nixon's "War on Cancer" in the 1970s produced important advances in molecular biology. Many of these discoveries proved invaluable as a basis for AIDS research in the 1980s. This research has in turn been responsible for significant contributions in virology, immunology, and microbiology. Increased understanding of gene expression, the immune system, viral evolution, and disease susceptibility are byproducts of AIDS research that are of great value, whether or not research ultimately leads to an AIDS vaccine or cure.[31]

Nor are annual mortality and morbidity rates necessarily the best way to assess health impact. By estimating the number of years of potential life lost (YPLL) to a particular hazard, an easily neglected sense of longer-term costs both to individuals and to society can be captured. By that measure, HIV infection, which claims a disproportionate share of persons in the prime of life, ranks as considerably more damaging than it would otherwise.[32] Charles Backstrom of the University of Minnesota and Leonard Robins of Roosevelt University noted, for example, that although AIDS is a small proportion of all deaths in Minnesota (which had a cumulative total of 840 cases by the end of 1990) it had become "the fifth leading cause of death among men aged twenty to sixty-four [in Minnesota]" and the leading cause of years lost by men in Minneapolis during 1989.[33] And even more than a decade after the discovery of AIDS, the future scale of victimization, particularly when considered in global perspective, remained uncertain.

The large increases in AIDS funding have not occurred consistently. Fiscal years 1983 to 1988 showed dramatic growth as a strong political constituency for AIDS funding developed.[34] Total NIH obligations for AIDS rose dramatically from $3,355,000 in fiscal year 1982 to $21,668,000 the following year, an increase of 546 percent in nominal dollars. From fiscal 1984 to fiscal 1988 yearly nominal dollar percentage increases were 104, 44, 111, 94, and 81, respectively. Then the rate of growth slowed to 27 percent in fiscal 1989, 23 percent in fiscal 1990, and slightly more than 8 percent in fiscal 1991.

By the late 1980s AIDS was widely perceived to have reached its fair share of budget dollars, inclining Congress toward smaller annual increments.[35] This shift was perhaps inevitable, as researchers and advocates concentrating on other diseases resisted AIDS-related funding increases that might imperil their own concerns. With the election of Bill Clinton, however, the balance once again tipped in favor of significant increases for AIDS. Public Health Service support for AIDS research shot up by about 18 percent to $1.5 billion for fiscal year 1994, with the NIH getting about $1.3 billion of that.[36]

While claims of excessive AIDS research funding might seem plausible, they remain unconvincing. To say how much is enough, subordinate questions must be addressed that inherently elude definitive answers. How much money will be required to find a cure or a safe and effective vaccine? How many more worthy research proposals can be generated? What value is placed on the lives and good health of those to be spared by making these benefits available? What value is placed on the potential alternative uses of the necessary funds? What larger or more distant applications might AIDS research have? Answers are elusive not only for technical reasons (that is, the necessary calculations are maddeningly difficult to make, assuming they can be made at all) but also for political ones.

Research and Its Management

A romantic image of science envisions the dedicated researcher bent over a microscope or test tube uncovering nature's secrets with a sudden flash of insight. These kinds of dramatic breakthroughs sometimes occur. In late 1976 the CDC's Joseph McDade looked through a microscope at a slide that had been examined months earlier and noticed the organism that caused Legionnaires' disease. In 1982 an observant Willy Burgdorfer of the NIAID dissected a deer tick collected on Shelter Island, New York. "In doing so," he later recounted, "I encountered in the midgut sluggishly moving microorganisms that I recognized as spirochetes."[37] In this way science learned, finally, how deer ticks transmit Lyme disease. And in 1984 researchers developed a test capable of detecting antibodies to HIV in the blood of infected persons.

Developments are not usually so dramatically positive. The reasons have less to do with heroism or negligence—though events are sometimes portrayed in this light—than with more mundane factors that are not easy to manage. Institutional structures, procedures, and priorities can do only so much to produce insight and creativity. One cannot simply mandate or reorganize to obtain knowledge. Pursuit of technology depends on solving both an incentive problem and a knowledge problem, and deliberate policy choices can far more easily influence the former than the latter.

The Incentive Problem

Adjusting the research agendas of NIH funders and scientists is not as simple as throwing a switch. The scientific enterprise is more self-contained and too complicated for that. Scientists settle on their individual research agendas for various reasons including intellectual interest, technical feasibility, and the desire for professional recognition. To sustain a career, research must prove fundable and yield publishable results. AIDS research was hampered for several years—some would contend that it remains so—by a dearth of researchers with the background and inclination to work on it. In the summer of 1990 the NIAID decided to create a new pool of cooperative agreement funds targeted at the HIV-related opportunistic infections, ailments that collectively inflicted the most immediate and visible harm on infected persons with badly damaged immune systems. The reason was that the existing drug discovery groups, which constituted the agency's primary commitment to preclinical drug development for AIDS, had at that time received not a single application to work on such infections. Some critics of the scientific establishment's response to AIDS have long maintained that such infections are inherently less appealing than HIV to professionally ambitious scientists.[38]

Similar problems confronted policymakers anxious to respond to the new threats of drug-resistant strains of tuberculosis and chronic fatigue syndrome. NIAID Director Anthony Fauci noted in congressional testimony that recent decades had seen few young investigators pursuing work on TB "because they did not see it as a problem, and for their own career development they did not see it as exciting enough or having enough visibility."[39] The elusive nature of CFS's causal mechanism combined with persistent skepticism about its validity as a genuine disease discouraged researchers from making the commitment to

work on it. By late 1991 hopeful observers believed that this was changing as an increased knowledge base persuaded more researchers that
the syndrome could be studied. "Success breeds success," Stephen E.
Straus, chief of the NIAID laboratory of clinical investigation, told the
journal *Science*. "When one shows that even an amorphous syndrome
like this is amenable to scrutiny—that you can generate reasonable
data out of it—other good people start feeling it's worthwhile to venture
into the field."[40] Criticizing scientists for selfishness or shortsightedness
does little good. Instead, contrary incentives must be offered, perhaps
through appropriately targeted cooperative agreements and contracts,
both of which allow much stronger NIH guidance and collaboration
than do grants.

The incentives of institutions matter as much as those of individuals,
with the former often driving or constraining the latter. To a degree
impossible to gauge precisely, efforts to produce AIDS drugs and vaccines have repeatedly confronted at least three versions of this problem,
all stemming from the powerful motivation of private firms to behave
in ways consistent with their financial interests. There exist in principle
strategies for coping with each.

One version derives from market size. Some diseases may afflict too
few persons to make investment attractive without a subsidy. (On
average, according to one study, it takes twelve years and $200 million
or more to get one new medicine from the laboratory to the pharmacist's
shelf.)[41] Well before recognition of the HIV epidemic, disease advocates
were lobbying Congress to create incentives for drug sponsors to
develop such "orphan drugs," resulting in the 1983 Orphan Drug Act.
A few AIDS drugs have held orphan drug status, though the sheer
scale of the epidemic has probably done more than anything else in
the long run to persuade firms to pursue that particular market.

A second version of the problem has to do with proprietary interest.
A firm might shy away from the investment required to manufacture
and market a drug if it feared underpricing by competitors who have
not had to bear similar costs. This is a potential problem where a drug
lies in the public domain, as AZT had in the years before the HIV
epidemic. Ultimately (and with much subsequent controversy over the
drug's stratospheric retail price) Burroughs Wellcome developed AZT,
which became the first, and highly unsatisfactory, antiviral therapy
approved to combat AIDS. The problem of proprietary interest has a

remedy in exclusive marketing rights, though this does not solve the problem of high prices faced by patients.

The third version of the problem is liability exposure. The search for AIDS drugs and vaccines has faced this hurdle repeatedly. In mid-1992 Abbott Laboratories postponed human trials of HIV hyperimmune globulin, a preparation that showed promise of preventing infected pregnant women from passing HIV to their children in the womb. Abbott had contracted with the NIH but wanted a liability waiver, which the agency did not have authority to grant.[42] Some scientists and potential AIDS vaccine manufacturers have also proved reluctant, particularly because vaccines, unlike therapies, must usually be given to healthy persons who might claim injury as a result.[43] This problem too has a solution, albeit a potentially expensive one: liability protection such as that offered swine flu vaccine manufacturers in 1976.[44]

The Knowledge Problem

Even when funding and research incentives do not pose special problems, creating precisely the knowledge sought remains problematic. An obvious point, perhaps, but it bears emphasis because naïveté about science and technology, and suspicion of those who produce them, are so common. (The latter is greater today than in eras when science commanded greater deference.) It is evident in the sometimes extreme rhetoric of AIDS activists and in the muckraking literature that has emerged about the epidemic.[45] Widely publicized accounts of scientific misconduct (including fraud and the unethical treatment of research subjects) enhance neither public confidence in science nor understanding of the serious and routine hurdles scientists face.[46]

Possible scandals and conspiracies aside, scientists are bound to approach problems with a different frame of mind than, say, patients with a stake in research outcomes. While the scientist and the activist or lobbyist may be on the same side in certain battles (funding, for example), the scientist grows nervous about encroachment by the layperson regarding the substance of research. Inevitably, tension arose between AIDS researchers accustomed to traditional research doctrine (including a reliance on lengthy placebo-controlled treatment trials and a reluctance to conflate research with mass treatment) and people with AIDS who have their own ideas about promising research avenues and demand sensitivity to their limited treatment options.[47] Similarly, when

Lyme disease patient-support groups sought to widen the definition of what constituted research worthy of consideration at a scientific meeting, a natural resistance arose among scientists.[48]

When attacking a new problem, prior interests and existing knowledge may prove crucial. The various ailments that became known collectively as AIDS fortunately appeared early to Gallo and his colleagues as possibly triggered by a retrovirus, an organism for which the NCI had been at the forefront of research. However, when the nation confronted an increase in tuberculosis, including a frightening surge in drug-resistant varieties of the TB bacillus, years of inattention to the organism's pathogenesis (the way it spreads in the body and produces disease) was one handicap repeatedly cited.[49] When an infectious disease appears or claims renewed interest, scientists may be poorly prepared to comprehend immediately the organism responsible (as with Legionnaires' disease and AIDS) or crucial specifics of organism-victim interaction (as with TSS, CFS, AIDS, and other illnesses).

Asked to imagine an ameliorative technology to defeat a serious infectious disease, the average person is inclined to "magic bullet" answers: a vaccine to prevent the disease or a treatment to cure it. But even when a problem is well publicized and made an explicit research priority, such technology is to a large extent hostage to complexities inherent in nature and scientists' uncertain grasp of its mechanisms and typically takes years to produce.

Although vaccine technology is rapidly advancing, one must keep in mind how few diseases are vaccine-preventable.[50] Though effective immunization dates back two centuries to Edward Jenner's pioneering success against smallpox, only about two dozen human diseases are currently susceptible to immunization—several of them public health milestones.[51] But for many infectious diseases of continuing importance—including syphilis, gonorrhea, and the common cold—no effective vaccine exists.

Once a vaccine is developed and licensed, its efficacy may be limited in ways difficult to predict or avoid. Though vaccines can be produced against particular strains of influenza, ongoing genetic variation undermines even the theoretical possibility of a single shot that would protect against all future infections. Moreover, influenza vaccine may not fully immunize a recipient. Disease may still occur, though it is less likely to be severe.[52] While critics often attributed the resurgence in measles cases during the 1980s to Reagan and Bush administration budget cuts that undermined the scope of immunization, the outbreaks often involved inadequately vaccinated children along with unvaccinated ones. Walter Orenstein, director of the CDC's division of immunization, told Congress in 1989 that a median of 60 percent of the measles cases occurring in outbreaks during 1985–86 had a history of vaccination. "Outbreaks have been reported in schools with 99 percent immunization levels and 96 percent immunity levels documented by laboratory tests," testified Orenstein. "Thus, the major problem appears to be that under some circumstances measles can be sustained among the 2 percent to 5 percent of vaccinees who fail to respond to an initial vaccination," a possibility that ultimately led most states to require a second shot.[53] The resurgence of tuberculosis in the late 1980s, including the sudden sharp rise in cases of deadly drug-resistant TB, occurred despite the availability of an immunizing agent, the Bacille Calmette-Guérin (BCG) vaccine. Use of BCG has been controversial in the health community, partly because of doubts about its effectiveness—some studies have found little or no efficacy, especially in adults—and partly because the vaccine undermines the standard TB skin test.[54]

A 1985 study by the Institute of Medicine neatly summarized many of the difficulties that have confronted vaccine innovation:

Identification of the causative organism is only the first step. The pathogenesis of the infection (how the organism produces the disease), what components of the organism are responsible for the manifestations of the disease (infectivity, virulence, pathogenicity) and which determine subsequent immunity, and whether current techniques can be anticipated to produce a safe and effective immunizing agent all represent crucial questions. The basic research necessary to answer these questions, which is often extremely time-consuming and expensive, usually is performed by investigators exploring the natural history of the disease. Commercial manufacturers rarely consider the possibility of a specific vaccine until the groundwork has been laid, typically by academic or government researchers.

The most basic technical requirement is the ability to consistently produce the organism (maintaining its immunogenicity) in the laboratory in sufficient quantities for study and, ultimately, for vaccine production. A reliable means must be found to measure immunity without exposure to disease. Researchers also must determine if the organism exists as more than one immunologically distinct type. For example, there are more than 80 immunologically distinct types of pneumococci, and infection or immunization with one type generally produces strong immunity only to that specific type.

Many questions depend on the nature of the organism. For example, in the case of an anticipated bacterial vaccine, can the immunity-producing component(s) be separated from irrelevant, potentially toxic moieties? Can the immunogenic antigen of a virus be extracted or, employing techniques of genetic engineering, be incorporated into another organism? In the case of a potential live vaccine, can the virulence of the pathogen be attenuated in the laboratory, and can reversion to the more virulent form be avoided with certainty?

The development of an animal model to evaluate toxicity, potency, and, if possible, clinical protection usually is desired. In addition, laboratory tests must be established, insofar as possible, to assess the toxicity and potency of the vaccine in a manner that correlates with test results in man.[55]

The search for both HIV and Lyme disease vaccines has had to confront such questions.[56] In 1990 Lyme disease researchers announced that they could immunize mice using an outer surface protein from the causal bacterium, *Borrelia burgdorferi*.[57] But the mice were challenged with the bacteria through injection. Would humans fare as well when encountering the bacteria through a tick bite? Some evidence suggested that "tick saliva may somehow enhance infectivity or that lab strains living couch-potato existences in culture plates may lack the vigor of wild-type bacteria."[58] Later research would indicate that vaccinated mice could withstand exposure to *Borrelia* through tick bites.[59] Yet researchers would still need to establish that a vaccine could protect against strains of the bacterium other than those found in laboratory-bred ticks. The lack of a good animal model posed a potential problem; some thought that expensive primate research might be necessary before a vaccine could be tried in humans.[60] By 1993 scientists were preparing for field trials of a promising vaccine that would employ the surface protein (instead of live or killed spirochetes).[61] This meant that a vaccine against Lyme disease would be widely available, at the earliest, two decades after the problem was first recognized.

Technical difficulties of a similar nature have also faced AIDS researchers, who could induce immunity to simian immunodeficiency virus (SIV) in the rhesus macaque, albeit under idealized and tightly controlled conditions. (Infection with SIV quickly kills rhesus macaques.) But chimpanzees, which offered a more favorable model in their ability to contract HIV, posed a problem: They did not, so far as anyone could tell, develop disease.[62] Researchers believed that they could protect chimps against HIV infection when challenged with free virus but then had to show that similar results might be obtained when HIV-infected white blood cells were employed. Results were encouraging but ambiguous.[63] Only in 1992, some eight years after the discovery of HIV, did scientists finally believe they had hit upon a good animal model for studying it and thus pursuing candidate vaccines; the pigtail macaque developed not only infection but also disease symptoms (though not full-blown AIDS).[64] Even so, HIV, like other microorganisms, comes in varieties or strains. HIV-1, the virus associated with disease in the United States, apparently clusters into recognizable families, each containing multiple strains.[65] An AIDS vaccine would have to cope with this variation.[66]

At the end of 1992 the press trumpeted a breakthrough said to offer "cautious hope," as a Washington Post headline put it, in the search for an AIDS vaccine.[67] Harvard researchers reported that six rhesus monkeys had been completely protected for three years against SIV. The vaccine employed contained live SIV with a key gene (called nef) removed. Could a similar procedure create a safe and effective human vaccine? Given enough time, perhaps so. But both Anthony Fauci and Robert Gallo expressed concern that removing nef might not permanently disable the virus. "The work is gorgeous. The [researchers are] very good," observed Gallo. "But the big question is, who would you want to try this vaccine on? Because if you ask me it's a big risk." Ronald Desrosiers, one of the researchers, predicted to the Post that, in light of the risks involved, a human vaccine would have to be evaluated for a decade or more, and even then might only be appropriate for people at a very high risk of contracting HIV. By the end of 1993 Science was reporting diminished hopes among HIV vaccine researchers.[68]

Predictably, the search for acellular pertussis vaccines went more smoothly. Scientific knowledge was much further developed for Bordetella pertussis, the causative microorganism, than for either Lyme disease or AIDS, the pathogens for which were isolated only in the 1980s. The pertussis microbe was first artificially cultivated in 1906, and a whole-cell vaccine was available before the outbreak of World War I.[69] Several currently exist, and an acellular vaccine was licensed in Japan as early as 1981.

Yet even the acellular pertussis vaccine exemplifies the problematic nature of research because the first two vaccines licensed in the United States, ACEL-IMUNE (marketed by Lederle Laboratories) and Tripedia (Connaught Laboratories) could not immediately address the core problem that vaccine skeptics claimed existed. The vaccines were initially approved by the FDA only for the fourth and fifth DPT booster shots, administered when a child is eighteen months and five to six years old. But the first three doses, given at two, four, and six months of age still consisted of whole-cell pertussis vaccine, and most allegations of serious vaccine injury have centered precisely on these pretoddlers.[70]

The limited approval stemmed from foreign data that made the FDA and the government's Advisory Committee on Immunization Practices cautious. "In Japan, with the continued use of acellular pertussis vaccines, the incidence of disease and death caused by pertussis has declined steadily," the committee noted. "However, the reported incidence among children age < 2 years has remained higher than the incidence among children of that age when whole-cell vaccines were routinely used in infants."[71] Although the vaccine advocacy group Dissatisfied Parents Together proclaimed itself pleased when the first acellular vaccine gained regulatory approval—"Anything is better than what we have now," commented a lawyer representing the group—the truth was that uncertainty embedded in research findings had, at that point at least, denied the group anything like a complete victory.[72] Whether an acellular vaccine could to be made available before the fourth dose was a question that only more data could answer.

Innovation in treatment is likewise problematic. When scientists are confronting an important new pathogen that is not self-limiting, such as HIV, they can screen the repertoire of existing therapies or make efforts to develop new ones.[73] Since the 1980s the NIH has screened tens of thousands of substances in the search for AIDS treatments, but the overwhelming majority have quickly proved useless. Some displayed anti-HIV activity in vitro but failed when tested in humans. Although a rumor-fed AIDS drug underground would develop, allowing desperate participants (with a benign nod from FDA regulators) to obtain unlicensed and untested drugs for their personal use, its main result was repeated disappointment.[74]

HIV is not the only elusive target for research intended to yield antiviral therapies. Antiviral drugs generally have emerged with agonizing slowness, largely because viruses, by definition, use a host to replicate, and identifying ways of interfering with viral replication that do not harm the host has proven difficult. A Pharmaceutical Manufacturers Association spokesperson observed in 1988 that only seven antivirals were available at that time, "compared to a couple of hundred anti-bacterial drugs." Four of the seven he listed were herpes treatments.[75] Charged with examining the general threat posed by emerging infections, a committee of the Institute of Medicine described the problem of antiviral therapy in pessimistic terms:

> Despite the efforts of researchers to discover new, effective antiviral drugs, very few ever reach the point at which they may become available to those who need them. Thousands of compounds may be screened before a single candidate with desirable antiviral properties and acceptable tolerance is found. Drugs that are potentially useful against viral infections fit into three categories: those that inactivate viruses (virucides); those that inhibit the replication of viruses within their host cells (antivirals); and those that work indirectly by augmenting or modifying the host's immune response to viral invasion (immunomodulators). . . . There are no clinically practical virucidal drugs at this time, since those currently available are toxic to host cells as well as viruses. Unlike those antibiotics that are bactericidal and can rid the patient of the organism, current antivirals only suppress viral replication. Ultimately, control of the viral infection relies on the individual's immune response.
>
> Antiviral drugs can interfere with viral invasion and replication at several specific points. For example, the drug can prevent the attachment of the virus to the host cell, or it may interfere with the assembly of new viruses within the host cell. Although many compounds that have antiviral activity exist or can be synthesized, most cannot be used because of toxicity, because they adversely affect a host cell function, or because they fail to reach concentrations required for antiviral activity in humans.[76]

Needed breakthroughs may also arrive slowly in the area of diagnostic testing. Treatment exists for Lyme disease, but efficacy is highest when the treatment is begun soon after infection. The symptoms of the disease are diverse; some 20 to 40 percent of infected persons never develop or never see erythema migrans, the distinctive circular rash that appears shortly after an infected tick bite.[77] Unfortunately, diagnostic tests for Lyme disease have proved notoriously unreliable, and a tedious search for good ones has frustrated health providers and disease advocates alike.[78] The lack of a sensitive test meant that Lyme disease would often be hardest to identify precisely when most vulnerable to treatment. A similar problem applies to MDR-TB. The several weeks needed to determine the pattern of drug susceptibility in a given patient meant that "suspicion of drug resistance on epidemiologic and clinical grounds [would] remain essential for the control of drug-resistant tuberculosis."[79]

Although political advocacy cannot create treatments and vaccines, it can transform institutional structure, procedure, and mindset. Ultimately, the NIAID's four divisions would include one devoted to AIDS, with NIAID Director Anthony Fauci wearing a second hat as NIH associate director for AIDS research when no other disease rated an associate directorship.[80] A decade into the epidemic found the NIH pursuing vaccines and therapies through eleven National Cooperative Vaccine Development Groups and twenty-eight National Cooperative Drug Discovery Groups—multi-institutional and multidisciplinary consortia focused on AIDS. The agency sponsored clinical trials of promising substances through nearly fifty institutions participating in the AIDS Clinical Trials Group (ACTG).[81]

Activists hurled perhaps their sharpest barbs at the traditional approach to clinical trials. Like other long-term and specialized endeavors, government-funded biomedical research has been the province of an establishment wedded to procedural and judgmental orthodoxies. Under the orthodox approach to clinical trials, only patients meeting certain carefully defined criteria could be admitted, and some of those might get inadequate treatment or a placebo, depending on the research protocol. Drugs have traditionally moved toward regulatory approval through three major, and often laborious, phases over a period of several years.

AIDS activists successfully challenged the status quo, pleading that people would die while scientists adhered to the traditional process. AIDS lobbying and activism pressured the research establishment to make AIDS a high priority and to be more flexible. The first meant more money, compatible with a traditional strategy of research proliferation. The second entailed departures from the reigning orthodoxy, resulting in the acceptance of efficacy data on aerosolized pentamidine gathered outside the usual channels and decisions to shorten and side-step traditional processes.[82] Even scientists who were not susceptible to direct pressure began to reexamine the orthodoxy, promoting creative ways to simplify, speed up, and enlarge clinical trials.[83] The 1990 enactment of the Ryan White CARE Act gave the linkage of research and mass treatment a legislative seal of approval, providing demonstration grants for research and services for pediatric AIDS in pursuit of both goals simultaneously.[84]

Most emergent public health hazards will not present difficulties in balancing urgency and restraint in biomedical research. For many problems, extensive research will be unnecessary or inappropriate. For others, restrained reaction and a relative lack of controversy will follow from the limited size, resources, objectives, and vehemence of the relevant disease constituencies. The Lyme Disease Foundation has a tiny staff (headquartered in Connecticut, not Washington) and a modest budget, and has mostly pursued restrained lobbying. Its leaders have eschewed dramatic hearings, accusatory public rhetoric, and big appropriations in favor of quiet contacts with scientists, government officials, and key members of Congress.[85] Both Lyme disease and chronic fatigue syndrome have spawned patient-support networks oriented far more toward distributing practical help to their members than publicly berating the government.[86] For both diseases, traditional low-profile advocacy supplemented by routine constituent contacts has served to sustain interest in the congressional appropriations subcommittees with jurisdiction over the NIH budget. For these diseases, total appropriations and aggregate political demand have been modest enough to obviate concerns of excessive priority skewing or research redundancy.

But even institutionalized urgency does not guarantee substantive success. Sophisticated observers understood long ago that the struggle to find effective antiretroviral therapies of tolerable toxicity would likely be arduous. A hard truth is that, despite enormous strides in understanding and taming viruses, a cure for viral disease remains unknown. Mostly, protective antibodies are stimulated through immunization or the body is allowed to cure itself.

These realities do not doom policy change to irrelevance, however. Critics accused the research establishment of insufficient concern with the opportunistic infections that kill so many HIV-infected persons. "Precious time was lost in the early years of the AIDS epidemic waiting for the discovery of a virus," wrote Mark Harrington of the ACT-UP treatment and data committee in a scathing 1990 critique of the ACTG program. "In the meantime, virtually no one in the upper echelons of U.S. biomedicine thought of going after the opportunistic infections."[87] Moreover, the ACTG had produced no new AIDS-related drugs. The NIH responded, with predictable defensiveness, that the ACTG had indeed sponsored valuable work on "28 agents for the prevention or treatment of OIs [opportunistic infections] and 12 cancer therapies" with considerable work forthcoming.[88] But even NIAID Director Fauci was clearly disappointed with the paucity of interest in opportunistic infections, which was why a national cooperative drug discovery group specifically targeted on such infections was announced not long after the Harrington critique.

In 1992 Harrington and Gregg Gonsalves, both of the newly formed Treatment Action Group (launched as an alternative to ACT-UP), stressed a deeper criticism. Government-sponsored research, they complained, was too virology-focused, insufficiently anchored in immunology, and moreover reflected inadequate coordination:

> OAR [the Office of AIDS Research] has no power to force the ICDs [institutes, centers, and divisions of the NIH] to do what they say they will; if they refuse to fund an AIDS program, OAR is helpless. Similarly the putative coordinating bodies such as the PHS AIDS Leadership Committee (ALC), the PHS Executive Task Force on AIDS (EFTA), or the AIDS Program Advisory Committee (APAC) lack information and power to coordinate the NIH's balkanized research projects. . . .
>
> The central questions of AIDS pathogenesis remain far from resolution after over a decade of research. The lack of attention to the immunopathogenesis of the disease, and the response of the host, reflect a larger problem in basic AIDS research: a general disregard for the physiological in basic research on the disease and the need to bridge the gap between basic and clinical research. While this may be heresy to some, pathogenesis research should look to the body for its future course; it needs a physiological and not simply an *in vitro* virology-driven foundation.[89]

A differently managed research effort during the 1980s might have produced additional or better drugs more quickly. But the argument that more and better drugs might have been available comes wrapped in an unspoken assumption: With more thoughtful and energetic management, they almost certainly would be. In 1993 hunger for institutional solutions led Congress to create a dramatically more powerful OAR, and HHS to announce a new National Task Force on AIDS Drug Development, intended to "identify and remove any barriers or obstacles to developing effective treatments," according to HHS Secretary Donna Shalala.[90] Casting a problem of fiendish technical difficulty in terms of plainly avoidable institutional failure risks making an unwarranted claim for even the most skillful research management.

Technical uncertainty aside, any rational and coordinated effort to make lots of drugs widely and quickly available must confront basic organizational incentives. Commercial drug sponsors hold stakes in specific products, not in drugs in general. Similarly, activists may have incentives to concentrate their effort on certain products, as when the Nation of Islam pushed for testing of oral alpha-interferon, also known as Kemron or Immuviron.[91] In other instances, products may simply seem particularly good candidates for quick approval. On occasion, commercial interests may also be tempted to employ raw political power. A major controversy erupted in 1992 when retired senator Russell B. Long, Democrat of Louisiana, who had chaired the Senate Finance Committee, successfully lobbied his former colleagues into approving $20 million for Defense Department research on gp160, a candidate AIDS "therapeutic vaccine" (that is, intended to boost the anti-HIV response of already infected persons instead of protecting the uninfected) sponsored by MicroGeneSys.[92] Scientists, including NIH Director Bernadine P. Healy, protested loudly and effectively that political clout was superseding scientific judgment.[93]

Conclusion

The greatest hurdle confronting those who would try to speed the availability of vaccines and treatments for AIDS, or anything else, is that the policy tools available (for example, research proliferation, abbreviated research, greater coordination, faster funding, faster dissemination of research results) cannot guarantee success, however creatively and assiduously implemented. This will remain true no matter how radically the scientific community redirects AIDS research in the years to come.[94] All that the NIH—as well as politicians, activists, drug companies, and university scientists—can do is take chances and offer incentives. The government may make informed guesses about the most promising avenues for inquiry and then "wave money in front of people" as one NIH middle manager put it, to entice enterprising scientists. Confronted with any major research goal toward which the agency wants to devote substantial extramural resources, the NIH must make the largest number of intelligent research bets possible with available resources. And intelligent bets are possible. The highly organized, interactive, and cumulative nature of modern science allows the agency a reasonable prospect of doing considerably better than a mere gambler, whose every roll of the dice is unaffected by previous rolls. But no one can reliably mandate development of complex technology when basic scientific understanding is lacking, no matter how high the public's anxiety or how strong the demand.

Eight

Prospects

THE EMERGENT public health hazard is a distressing, even frightening, phenomenon. Three general observations can help offset Andromeda strain—an excessive preoccupation with very unlikely sudden calamities.

First, even allowing for underreporting, many emergent health hazards have proved to be deadly but limited problems. The 1976 Legionnaires' disease outbreak, the Tylenol scare, the tainted L-tryptophan, and the 1993 outbreak of hantavirus pulmonary syndrome in the southwestern United States led to massive press coverage but fewer than 100 reported deaths nationally. A vigorous investigative and regulatory response by health officials quickly renders most such events containable tragedies. Some multisource infectious diseases are much harder to cope with (for example, AIDS, Lyme disease, and TB), but even these are preventable and are unlikely to afflict more than small fractions of the U.S. population.

Second, for the foreseeable future, familiar and less dramatic killers—cancer, heart disease, hypertension, injuries—will continue to dwarf the impact of most novel hazards by several orders of magnitude. This means that familiar and undramatic behavioral improvements—safe driving, reduced smoking, sensible eating, moderate drinking, regular exercise—will save and improve far more lives than high-profile efforts against new diseases.

Third, the United States has scored impressive, even dramatic, public health successes. Performance is admittedly uneven on some indicators, such as immunization rates and infant mortality. But overall, the combined effects of sanitation, antibiotics, and vaccines have produced changes inconceivable before the turn of the century, when fevers and sore throats routinely meant death in early childhood and when soldiers faced a greater risk of death from disease than from enemy ordnance. Also, despite considerable anxiety and public debate, catastrophes stemming from civilian technology have been notably scarce.[1] Moreover, many products (and especially newly developed ones that are injected, ingested, or implanted) must undergo rigorous testing for both safety and efficacy before marketing. (Cigarettes, an old and politically protected product, could never have cleared the existing regulatory barriers that apply to new drugs, food additives, and medical devices. But even smoking has dramatically declined since the 1950s.)[2] When a novel acute hazard strikes, mechanisms are in place to recognize and mobilize against it, and public health officials can institute ad hoc surveillance for a new ailment very rapidly.

Innumerable public health challenges remain, and not solely among persons of low income. Affluence and innovation regularly create new threats. Important infectious diseases can still appear, mutate, and migrate unpredictably.[3] Changes in life-styles (that is, in patterns of residence, travel, sexual activity, and so forth) may expose new populations to unexpected dangers, such as HIV or the spirochete that causes Lyme disease.[4] Medicines and medical devices may suddenly reveal unforeseen side-effects and vulnerabilities. Alternatively, drug and device problems previously known or suspected may become more broadly salient—as with silicone breast implants. Disease expected to be a serious problem may remain benign, even dormant (such as swine flu in 1976), for reasons about which specialists can only speculate. Inattention and increased microbial resistance to drugs may transform diseases once thought manageable (such as malaria, measles, or tuberculosis) into graver threats.[5] Aaron Wildavsky is undoubtedly right that "richer is safer," though largely because wealth can be used to purchase regulatory and other precautions.[6] The creation of overall wealth does not address either the unmet needs of the disadvantaged or the true costs of a bountiful modern life. Antibiotics are so widely available that they invite misuse leading to microbial resistance. A recent essay observed that, "from the public health perspective, uncompleted treatment [of TB] poses a greater threat than nontreatment" because the former facilitates MDR-TB.[7] Faster dissemination of influenza via "jetspread" or of tick-borne disease through suburban expansion into wooded areas is no less authentic simply because commercial air travel and suburbs are acknowledged as beneficial.[8] Similarly, fast food is here to stay but brings with it new possibilities for the mass consumption of bacteria-contaminated hamburger.[9]

Emergent public health hazards vary widely in technical complexity and in their prospects for quick policy consensus. Relatively easy problems include products that can be either temporarily or permanently removed from the marketplace, ideally with less hazardous substitutes remaining. Outbreaks of communicable disease are manageable to the extent that they are familiar, or similar to things that are, and associated with specific locales or practices amenable to previously successful intervention strategies. When a product causing acute harm can be neither withdrawn nor quickly reformulated, successful risk management becomes much more problematic—a matter of encouraging wise use. (Product withdrawal is also undermined when manufacturers shirk their responsibilities.) AIDS has likewise proved challenging on purely technical grounds. It was tough to identify initially, persistent in infected persons, resistant to known therapies, and transmitted in settings that are often impossible to regulate. Additionally, AIDS policy has been punctuated by concerns having little to do with disease control. For certain hazards institutions may be inclined to resist, or individuals to disregard, preventive efforts. Reye's syndrome and toxic shock syndrome are in the first category; MDR-TB, the second; and AIDS notably in both. Federal health agencies can respond aggressively to, but do not control, these dynamics. The more durable a threat is, the more likely it is to acquire policy complications, provoking dissatisfaction among those attentive to agency performance. The government's 1993 investigative response to an outbreak of rodent-borne hantavirus infection was generally lauded as a public health success.[10] The luster would fade, however, should hantavirus pulmonary syndrome cause a steeply rising death toll or should intervention run afoul of an organized constituency, such as the Navahos on whose land the outbreak occurred.

Limits of Anticipation

Emergent public health hazards need to be taken seriously, keeping their larger context and thorny realities in mind. Consideration might begin with Wildavsky's distinction between anticipation and resilience, two different but compatible approaches to hazards generally.[11] Anticipation attempts "to predict and prevent potential dangers before damage is done," while resilience involves "the capacity to cope with unanticipated dangers after they have become manifest, learning to bounce back."[12] Wildavsky argued that anticipation is the preferred course to the extent that danger emanates from foreseeable sources against which early intervention is feasible. (An example might be the surge in volcanic activity that clearly heralds a potentially devastating eruption. Anticipatory evacuation would be warranted.) Unfortunately, conditions usually do not favor precise anticipation. And guessing about a complex array of future hazards under conditions of uncertainty presents its own dangers. Advised Wildavsky: "In addition to the cost of using up society's resources on false leads—that is, leaving insufficient resources to counter unexpected dangers—each preventive program contains its own pitfalls."[13] Immunization may, for example, inadvertently victimize, as in the swine flu episode.

In one sense, anticipation and resilience are not only compatible but also inseparable. The process of bouncing back from specific troubles unavoidably and logically inspires efforts aimed at forestalling an identical recurrence as well as a different albeit similar problem. Were this not true, much meaningful learning would not occur. Experience with past product recalls, for example, informs later ones. Lessons absorbed during an immunization or educational campaign against a disease (mingled with reasonable anticipatory leaps of the imagination) will inspire subsequent efforts against other diseases. An outbreak of acute illness caused by *E. coli* in hamburger calls forth broader reforms to deal with various pathogens in meat generally. A particular brand of infant formula harboring a specific nutritional deficiency leads to the Infant Formula Act, intended to prevent a wide variety of deficiencies. An outbreak of diarrheal disease in Milwaukee lends additional impetus to a General Accounting Office study broadly criticizing state inspections of local water supplies.[14] The pattern is an old one. In major drug regulatory reforms of 1938 and 1962, and in response to the 1955 Cutter incident, hazards that were novel, serious, and suddenly apparent triggered a forward-looking reassessment of the policy status quo.[15] In this sense, anticipation and resilience are inextricably linked.

But accurate prediction is usually impossible. It is hard both to know the future and to motivate cooperation on the basis of what is presumably known. If hazardous products or batches could be identified beforehand, action would be taken to avoid victimization. That is not always possible.[16] Certain reforms (for example, more frequent inspections, toughened standards of premarket approval) will doubt-less prevent some problems that would otherwise arise, but their costs and limitations can be formidable. Absent a rapidly growing budget for regulatory bureaucracies, resource shifts driven by anticipatory maneuvers will leave other things less well scrutinized. And potentially useful products should not remain snared in regulatory proceedings unnecessarily. New infectious disease is at least as tough to anticipate as new product hazards. Where or when a new infectious disease will emerge cannot be known. And recognizing that a disease exists is different from having reliable information about when, or if, it might strike some specific locale. Like many sudden disasters, the Milwaukee cryptosporidiosis outbreak that affected an estimated 370,000 persons may have been the proverbial accident waiting to happen, and yet no one specifically predicted it even though implementation of the 1974 Safe Drinking Water Act was known to be glacial virtually everywhere.[17]

Where a preexisting stake in denying or downplaying risk prevails, support for anticipatory change will be correspondingly hard to mobilize. The AIDS epidemic offers the most tragic and visible example. Until the early 1980s health-related reservations about sexual promiscuity went largely unheeded by much of the gay community.[18] Some of the specific interpersonal behaviors that launched the epidemic in the United States are unsanitary and were known to be so long before AIDS appeared in 1980–81. By the mid-1970s homosexual men were displaying very high rates of previous exposure to hepatitis B virus, a far more infectious pathogen than HIV would turn out to be.[19] This generated little panic at the time, largely because infected men tended to recover from their bouts of acute illness.[20] A plethora of other sexually transmitted ailments, susceptible in most cases to antibiotics, were common among gay men as well. Given the gay community's anxiety about sexual freedom, a program of vigorous anticipatory warnings about a possible new lethal infection would likely have been widely ignored or openly derided, at least until people began to fall ill and die. (Even when the death toll began to mount, denial persisted for some time.) Nor would injecting drug users likely have rallied to a call for changed behavior that was unvalidated by street-level experience and frightening word of mouth about real victims, even though needle-borne epidemics are not new.[21]

Economic interests and comfortable consumers display a similar tendency. In the early years of the AIDS epidemic, gay bathhouses fought closure and blood banks resisted aggressive donor screening. In the same way, aviation accidents are often required to motivate industry reform of practices that had previously seemed acceptable risks, an inclination to which one commentator attached the grim label "blood response."[22] Qualms about the antibiotic-laced animal feeds that enhance livestock production have fared poorly in the political process. Hypothetical arguments about an exacerbated potential for antibiotic resistance are simply uncompelling when stacked against the immediate and visible benefits of such feeds.[23] Fierce business and consumer opposition erupted in 1977 when the FDA proposed to ban saccharin after a Canadian study indicated possible carcinogenicity.[24] Lacking tangible evidence of victimization, Congress quickly acted to ensure that protesting dieters and diabetics would have uninterrupted access to saccharin while more data were gathered (a political decision that turned out to have been reasonable on health grounds as well). Similarly, the lack of a major outbreak, as opposed to sporadic cases, of salmonella infection attributable to the consumption of certified raw (that is, unpasteurized) milk undermined efforts to withdraw the product from intrastate commerce during the 1980s.[25] While infectious disease specialists believed that they had amply documented the health risks, "the raw milk industry . . . stressed . . . [its] benefits . . . and minimized or denied any infectious disease hazards," abetted by raw milk advocates who believed it superior to the pasteurized product.[26] Neither antibiotic overuse nor any particular emerging infection is likely to receive much concentrated public attention or political interest until it victimizes concretely—and perhaps not even then. A 1994 CDC proposal for enhancing the nation's capability to address emerging infectious diseases points out that "both E. coli 0157:H7 and Cryptosporidium were first recognized as significant human pathogens in the early 1980s, but neither has received adequate public health attention."[27] Where regulatory action is visibly inconvenient or costly for an established interest, a cluster of victims is required before a problem is recognized as worth addressing. Identifiable victims allow for the true character of a threat to be grasped and generate a consensus for action. But resistance may remain even after all this has happened.

Prospects for Resilience

Because anticipation is so problematic, effective resilience—reaction continually modified by experience and new understanding—remains the practical goal for managing emergent hazards. History indicates where the likeliest successes will come: emergency investigations of acute disease (especially common-source epidemics) along with certain easy regulatory problems. At the other end of the spectrum, some intervention initiatives will be vigorously contested, and biomedical science, although vital and mostly noncontroversial over the long run, offers exceedingly unpredictable help, especially in the short run. A primary reliance on reaction need not mean leaving one's guard down completely until the first punch is delivered. The best prospects for fast response exist when the structures or practices that make it possible have been carefully and thoughtfully put in place.

Attempted resilience can go awry in numerous ways, but with two essential results: overreaction and underreaction. Once victimization becomes apparent, conclusions about its likely scope can be drawn that later turn out to have been unwarranted. For example, many exaggerated warnings were heard over the years about HIV spreading like wildfire among non-drug-using heterosexuals in the United States.[28]

The swine flu debacle of 1976 is the leading cautionary example of aggressive resilience.[29] In their highly critical study, political scientist Richard E. Neustadt and public health expert Harvey V. Fineberg concluded that the government overreacted by making too many premature decisions and wedding itself early to a course of action that did not adequately provide for subsequent contingencies and reappraisals.[30] Even if no institutional inadequacies or complexities had to be considered, the nature of influenza itself demanded caution; it is a particularly "slippery" disease, subject to many technical uncertainties.[31] One might reply that it is better to be safe than sorry when calamity threatens, but the potential price is high. False alarms can endanger institutional credibility and confidence, and thus undermine later resilience.

And yet, underreaction, the product of an inadequate institutional and public sense of urgency, is far more likely than insufficient restraint. The sources of underreaction—the difficulty of energizing and coordinating large, complex, and politically sensitive institutions; comfort with orthodox procedures and perspectives that have served well in the past; personal unwillingness to forgo known benefits or to take risks—are more likely present than forward-looking policy advocacy or quick receptivity to new approaches and agendas. This was a primary difficulty facing government officials shifting gears to cope with AIDS. The prompt recognition and investigation of novel acute hazards does not extend to complex interventions or to the realm of biomedical science. Some commentators have suggested that CDC Director David Sencer's experience with swine flu made him especially reluctant later when, as the local health commissioner, he oversaw New York City's early and tepid response to AIDS.[32]

Circumstances beyond centralized control largely determine government capacity to be resilient against emergent public health hazards. Federal agencies are powerfully constrained by the nature of the hazard and by the social and political context each presents, a context that varies across stages of response. The investigation of a disease is unlikely to be politicized, but later regulatory action relating to the same hazard may display the intense "operating room politics" of a highly salient and technically complex issue.[33] Were the Lyme spirochete an invariably fatal pathogen, or casually communicable among humans, or sexually transmitted, the politics of the disease would vastly differ, as would the prospects for mounting an effective response. If it displayed one or more of these characteristics, Lyme disease would claim a far higher priority and intense media interest, its victims perhaps stigmatized, and health officials subject to far more intense criticism. The social construction of disease is inescapable. Response will inevitably reflect how victims and their illnesses are perceived by the larger society, how the burdens of intervention are distributed, and the extent to which political organization is brought to bear. A disease that appears to focus on persons who are both organizable and stigmatized, as did AIDS initially, is bound to take a special political course that policymakers will be at pains to grapple with. If HIV caused death within hours or days of infection, ACT-UP could not exist, and there would be little need for it, partly because AIDS would far more quickly have riveted official attention and partly because the disease would probably have burned itself out within a comparatively short time.[34]

Two different, but not inconsistent, approaches exist to improve resilience. Generalized preparation allows resources to be deployed in advance of any specific threat to facilitate an effective reaction when one is needed. A more common means is focused reaction: revising a system either incrementally or radically once a specific threat is at hand and evolving.

Generalized Preparation

Three preparatory measures deserve attention. First is dramatically enhanced surveillance—the installation and operation of more or more sensitive tripwires to facilitate early detection and careful evaluation of an emerging hazard. This elicits little controversy, has considerable long-term practical significance, and so justifiably appeals to both the CDC and the FDA. To further encourage health professionals to notify the FDA of adverse events, the agency launched MEDWATCH, a program of streamlined voluntary medical products reporting, in June 1993.[35] Five different forms were consolidated into one, accompanied by a single mailing address, a fax number, and distribution of a new *FDA Desk Guide for Adverse Event and Product Problem Reporting*. But MEDWATCH lacks an independent means to assess reporting accuracy, a problem that helped lead Raymond L. Woosley, chairman of the department of pharmacology at Georgetown University Medical Center, to call for the creation of federally funded centers for education and research in therapeutics (CERTs). Woosley argues that such centers could independently assure the accuracy of adverse experience reports, promote physician compliance with the voluntary reporting system, and conduct research to identify rare adverse reactions to drugs.[36] Such centers might help raise the now low percentage of adverse reactions reported. They would also provide doctors with a source of information independent of a pharmaceutical industry that spends some $10 billion per year promoting drugs to physicians.

Dissatisfaction with the existing system of detecting infectious disease has led the CDC to develop an ambitious set of integrated proposals not only to improve monitoring and response by state and local agencies but also to facilitate more effective global surveillance.[37] Though anticipatory in tone, the CDC proposals would undergird resilience by relaying important information about the nature of epidemics to public health officials. The idea of strengthened national and global surveillance is an outgrowth of the renewed prominence accorded infectious disease since 1980, and especially since 1990. AIDS, resurgent TB, Lyme disease, and other more limited (or less publicized) disease outbreaks have helped motivate the CDC and the larger community of infectious disease specialists to pinpoint the inadequacies of the existing arrangements. A stronger surveillance infrastructure would facilitate response to the large majority of significant diseases for which the states receive no federal surveillance funds.[38] The ultimate impact on the course of new and newly recognized diseases is less certain because recognition does not equal effective intervention. Edwin D. Kilbourne of the Mount Sinai School of Medicine pointed out that existing global surveillance effectively discerns influenza virus mutations but that this knowledge "has not yet significantly altered the impact of the disease. . . . Surveillance for the unknown will be even more difficult and will demand a level of clinical and laboratory competence not widely available in the third world, or, for that matter, anywhere else."[39] Nevertheless, because any intervention first requires that a specific problem and its characteristics be identified, surveillance remains a cornerstone of response to all future public health hazards, the key to moving beyond theoretical possibilities to practical action.

A second and perhaps more familiar preparation is contingency funding. Reacting to several emergent hazards, including AIDS, the Tylenol poisonings, and the infant formula scare, Congress amended the Public Health Service Act in 1983 to authorize $30 million as a Public Health Emergency Fund, available when "a disease or disorder presents a public health emergency" or when "a public health emergency otherwise exists and the [federal government] has the authority to take action with respect to such emergency."[40] Congress cleared the legislation over the Reagan administration's objection. Assistant Secretary for Health Edward Brandt claimed that such a fund was unnecessary and argued instead for a much smaller ($5 million) allocation solely for the FDA.[41] Intended to facilitate response to sudden emergencies by reducing damaging raids on existing routines and priorities, contingency funding evokes restrained enthusiasm among congressional appropriators, who generally prefer that agencies either reprogram existing funds or request supplemental appropriations. Congress did not appropriate any money for the emergency fund, prompting the complaint that the legislation amounted to "a public relations ploy, not public health policy."[42] For the FDA, appropriators have followed the less generous path embraced by Assistant Secretary Brandt for the FDA, setting aside a modest contingency fund (about $4 million) on which it has drawn to handle, among other things, the L-tryptophan emergency.[43] Congress has been somewhat more generous to the NIH. Beginning in fiscal year 1991, it allowed the agency director a discretionary fund and authority to reallocate up to 1 percent of the total agency budget.[44] Under NIH Director Bernadine Healy, the money mainly supported Shannon Awards, grants for deserving extramural scientists whose work would otherwise have barely missed funding because of budget constraints even though peer reviewers judged it meritorious.[45]

Arguing that contingency funding facilitates the functioning of federal agencies is easier than showing that it promotes superior public health. Many hazards have required agencies to reallocate resources aggressively and quickly, a painful process.[46] But to claim that this makes a major substantive difference in the outcome of emergency response efforts, it must be shown how essential resources that would otherwise be brought to bear are forgone entirely and how emergencies therefore last longer, or spread farther, than a contingency funding mechanism would allow. With the possible exception of the AIDS epidemic, this would be hard to demonstrate. If such funding could be shown to have allowed product recalls or outbreak investigations that otherwise would not have occurred, the case for contingency funding would be especially strong. But supporters have offered no evidence of this for emergent public health hazards. And because these activities are central to the missions of the FDA and the CDC, a special pot of money is not needed to entice the agencies into attending to them. In this respect, the NIH would seem a more reasonable candidate for contingency funding, because sudden public health emergencies are historically more tangential to its core activities. But in light of the uncertainties that bedevil biomedical research, knowing in advance whether positive public health outcomes will ensue from the use of such a fund is impossible.

Contingency funding would make a substantive difference to the extent that it gave officials access to, or control over, money that would otherwise be unavailable for an emergency. In the case of product recalls particularly, most unbudgeted expenditures will be relatively small. In congressional testimony, an FDA official cited the figures $334,000 for the infant formula recall and $531,000 for the Tylenol scare.[47] Expenses can run into the millions of dollars, as they apparently did for the CDC in handling Legionnaires' disease and toxic shock syndrome.[48] But in the end, except for an unusually costly and complex emergency such as the AIDS epidemic, contingency funding is more likely to compensate an agency for unexpected expenditures than to make such expenditures possible in the first place. And given both a pervasive budget constraint and traditional inclination, congressional appropriators will be reluctant to bestow a large sum of money (say,

$50 million or $100 million) on the FDA or the CDC in anticipation of "the next AIDS."

A third generalized preparation has also been debated over many years: stronger market withdrawal authority for the FDA. The agency has long been able to get along without it. When it seeks the withdrawal of a product, the FDA must either go to court or prod the offending manufacturer into commencing a recall. But this particular balance of regulatory power may be altered. As supporters of a bolstered FDA emphasize, Congress has granted newer agencies (including the National Highway Traffic Safety Administration and the Consumer Product Safety Commission) the authority to order recalls.[49] But recent efforts to strengthen the FDA's field enforcement authority have proved politically contentious, stirring particular opposition from food industry lobbies.[50] Opponents argue that the agency has sufficient power already, and they conjure fears of an FDA unfairly playing the roles of judge, jury, and executioner. Given a choice between stronger enforcement authority and an infusion of material resources, FDA leadership would almost certainly choose the latter as far more helpful.[51] It is plausible that, as with contingency funding, unilateral recall authority might allow the FDA to handle episodes less stressfully but without significantly improved results to show for it. In any case, political opposition seems unlikely to abate soon.

Focused Reaction

What is largely left, then, is reacting to specific concretely manifested problems. Though this is by far the more common and familiar path, it does not inevitably lead to conventional responses. Focused reaction may be radical.

The special demands and frustrations of the AIDS epidemic inspired significant centralizing and decentralizing changes simultaneously. In the latter vein, the federal government was prodded by grass-roots activism toward acknowledgment and support of community-based research and toward greater formal and informal participation in decisionmaking by people with AIDS. Meanwhile, desires for strengthened coordination produced a PHS national AIDS program office, later the designation of Anthony Fauci as NIH associate director for AIDS research, and then in June 1993 the appointment of a White House AIDS policy coordinator (or AIDS czar) and legislation creating an enhanced office of AIDS research inside the NIH.[52] In 1991 the National

Commission on AIDS recommended that "a comprehensive national HIV plan should be developed with the full participation of involved federal agencies and with input from national organizations representing various levels of government to identify priorities and resources necessary for preventing and treating HIV disease."[53] To oversee the effort, the commission supported the assignment of a powerful coordinating entity:

> To develop the comprehensive national HIV plan, the Commission calls upon the President of the United States to designate an individual or lead agency with the authority and responsibility for instituting a cabinet-level process to articulate the federal component of an HIV plan, develop a mechanism for interagency as well as state and local participation and coordination, and establish a timeline for completion of key tasks.[54]

At least as ambitious, and more controversial, is a so-called Manhattan Project for AIDS. Employed by candidate Bill Clinton during the 1992 presidential campaign, and deliberately conjuring up the secret crash program that developed the atomic bomb, the term has been embraced by some activists and scientists, though what precisely they intend is conflicting or unclear.[55] The most radical versions envision a coordinated program of directed research operating outside the traditional NIH apparatus to answer lingering questions blocking the path to effective treatments and vaccines.

As a targeted response to the AIDS epidemic, dramatically heightened federal coordination remains exceedingly problematic. The many specific problems associated with AIDS boil down to two for which policy coordination is an inherently weak tool: limited knowledge and political disagreement.[56]

As of 1994 scientists still do not know how to kill or neutralize HIV once introduced into the bloodstream of a human host. Also undetermined is how confidently to induce and sustain in targeted populations the personal preventive behaviors that inhibit the introduction of HIV. No administrative mechanism, whether centered in the NIH or the Oval Office, can dependably create the research breakthroughs or insights into human behavior required to overcome these essential scientific hurdles that AIDS poses. Virtually everybody has heard that smoking cigarettes, driving while intoxicated or without a seat belt, injecting illegal drugs, and eating lots of saturated fat are undesirable.

But varying fractions of the population will do all of these things regardless of the government's efforts to prohibit or advise against them.

The point is not that a tightly focused or carefully coordinated search for effective interventions would be either impossible or ineffective. More is learned about AIDS and HIV every day, and interorganizational cooperation of various kinds and at many levels is often crucial to progress. Nor have all promising paths toward vaccines and therapies been taken. Activists who chastise the government for, among other things, too much virology and not enough immunology deserve to be heard. And to the extent that ambitious scientists can be induced to pursue a common agenda of filling gaps in existing knowledge, an important hurdle will have been overcome.

But even if the traditional belief is dismissed that centralized direction of research is less likely to be productive than investigator-driven science, no way exists to be certain in advance which particular administrative or budgetary arrangements, and in which combinations, are most likely to unravel key mysteries or what kind of leadership would be best able to make critical judgments about priorities at precisely the right points. As appealing as the sound of creating a coordinated effort to combat AIDS is, assuming it could be akin to the Manhattan Project is a mistake. All relevant brainpower could not be relocated at one facility, and AIDS activists would never tolerate either the secrecy or the dictatorial management that nurtured the atomic bomb project. When the atomic bomb facility began operating at Los Alamos, New Mexico, in 1943, its leaders could be reasonably certain that a weapon was attainable soon given enough resources; a reliable scientific theory predicted that nuclear fission, properly triggered, would yield an explosion of unprecedented power. Several crucial hurdles—devising a detonator, producing enough fissionable material, calculating the most efficient configuration of that material, and so on—were largely problems of technology, of inspired engineering, instead of the basic science that has hobbled progress against AIDS.[57] Los Alamos scientists never faced the equivalent of viral replication or mutation, or arduous clinical trials involving potentially uncooperative research subjects. A dozen years into the AIDS epidemic, a review in the *New England Journal of Medicine* began by stating that "the human immunodeficiency virus . . . is probably the most intensively studied virus in the history of biomedical research" and concluded with the sobering observation that the "immunopathogenic mechanisms of HIV infection are complex and not well understood."[58]

The term *coordination* is itself misleading to the extent that political persuasion is the real heart of the matter. The difficult AIDS issues of condom distribution, needle exchange programs, and treatment funding do not provoke misunderstandings or administrative confusion that could be rectified with a few good meetings. Instead, real policy disagreements grounded in moral claims and competing priorities exist. Early and laudably, the Clinton administration urged Congress to offer far more money for local treatment services under the 1990 Ryan White CARE Act than the Bush administration had. But this was a hard political choice, not coordination. Many Americans so abhor homosexual conduct, illegal drug use, and sexual relations among unmarried minors that they recoil from even potentially life-saving policies that suggest a validation of these activities or expose their families to a discussion of them. Needle exchange is a promising idea that some communities have productively supported but that many persons (including liberals) approach warily.[59] Anyone, whether White House policy coordinator or president, trying to calm these troubled waters through mere coordination faces an impossible job.

Perhaps the most radical and breathtakingly comprehensive vision yet offered for coping with AIDS was inspired by another legendary success: the Polaris missile program that created the first submarine-launched nuclear weapon.[60] Sociologists Charles Perrow and Mauro F. Guillén borrow from this experience (described in detail by MIT political scientist Harvey M. Sapolsky) to recommend an all-out war, a "crusade" against AIDS.[61] Operating from a Special Projects Office inside the Navy, the Polaris program of the 1950s spared no expense, had priority over virtually all other competing needs, and was sold relentlessly and effectively as essential to keeping communism at bay. As Perrow and Guillén recounted:

> The program to do what no one had done before was sold to the nation, to the contractors, and to the navy personnel involved as a crusade. The danger of Communist invasion was less imminent and less predictable than the danger of AIDS, but forces enlisted to combat the threat were invested with a religious fervor. Daily briefings started with prayer meetings, and the wives of personnel were urged to sacrifice their home life for the safety of the country. Funds

were to be ample; no part of the program could suffer because of lack of money. Congress caught the spirit too, twice voting hundreds of millions more in funds than President Eisenhower's White House asked for. Military contractors, Sapolsky noted, were able to satisfy long standing 'wish lists' for equipment and projects that were unrelated to the program. This was not called corruption or favoritism. The technology was uncertain; no existing programs had been proven efficient. Therefore eleven different launching systems were worked on at once, and the redundant ones were simply abandoned when a decision was made. No one complained of inefficiency. If underwater launches could not be achieved, surface launches would be sufficient—the goals were realistic even if the passionate desired [the infeasible]. If a component failed a test, no inquiry was made into the reason for the failure; that would delay progress. Instead, contracts were let for alternative designs of the component, and each design was tried until one worked.[62]

Were the public convinced that the AIDS epidemic might destroy the country or change everyday life intolerably, one can imagine a no-holds-barred program of this sort being put into place. Members of Congress might be seen on television handing out clean needles, with the president having long ago issued a resounding call to condoms and maybe even mandatory testing. But the country is not so persuaded, nor should it be. While AIDS has ravaged certain stigmatized and disadvantaged groups in the United States, the larger society thus far does not appear threatened.[63] In light of this, resource constraints and political disagreement remain for AIDS policy. Prospects for the political system's acceptance of poor accounting, fraud, or apparent waste for the sake of defeating AIDS seem dim; journalists and politicians remain poised to cast blame on precisely these grounds.[64] A far more promising and politically viable approach would entail concentrating preventive effort on the relatively small number of identifiable neighborhoods in twenty-five to thirty cities where HIV infection and transmission rates are highest.[65] This could be done—and would have to be done—without addressing comprehensively the "root causes" (that is, poverty, hopelessness, and so on) against which liberals reflexively campaign.[66] But a frankness of language and a willingness to try the unorthodox (such as needle exchanges) will be required and will make many conservatives wince.

Perhaps the toughest question that emergent public health hazards present is not how to recognize a new problem but how to ensure that an authentic world-class disaster is quickly distinguishable from the many smaller and more manageable emergencies, many of which briefly seize attention before moving offstage. In preparing for the future, seeking villains retrospectively among persons whose behavior could not plausibly have been very different during the AIDS epidemic is not helpful. In hindsight, if Ronald Reagan's White House staff had prodded him successfully to take aggressive action against AIDS in 1981–82, the world would have been done an inestimable service. But this would also have violated the prime directive of White House staff: protect at all costs the personal and political interests of the president. Reagan wanted to reduce domestic spending and keep conservative support. Meanwhile, senior HHS officials pleaded for additional funding behind the scenes, while claiming publicly that they had sufficient resources, behavior that Perrow and Guillén label a "deception."[67] But officials are driven to such behavior by a system that demands both responsiveness and loyalty to the president's program. Had Jimmy Carter won reelection in 1980, the CDC would have had an old friend in the White House; Carter had been governor of Georgia, where the agency is headquartered. But regardless of who occupied the White House in the early 1980s, his intentions toward homosexuals, or his broader agenda, a major and deadly AIDS epidemic was unavoidable given the silent spread of infection for years before alarm bells started ringing.[68]

A more energetic and well-funded program of surveillance would provide the best chance to sound those alarms right away and to respond appropriately. And because neither the creation nor operation of surveillance infrastructure invites much controversy, this ought to be a preparatory reform that both liberals and conservatives can support. The main political problem facing such reform is less likely to be principled opposition than a simple indifference born of competing priorities and, ironically, the reputation that public health officials (especially the CDC) enjoy for successfully recognizing and investigating new problems. Public health authorities have begun to articulate a strong technical case for improved surveillance capacities, but the political case may be less compelling. As with policymaking for AIDS, the active support of senior federal health officials, and perhaps the president, could make a major political difference.

Notes

Chapter One

1. Some might question whether AIDS has any real near-term impact on persons infected with HIV, because the estimated mean is eight to ten years between infection and the development of symptomatic AIDS. Two responses may be offered. The first is that, once detected, even asymptomatic HIV infection victimizes through social stigma and psychological impact. Second, the estimated mean is only that; many infected persons develop AIDS much more rapidly. The connection between HIV and AIDS is not comparable to the more distant and tenuous link between, for example, radiation exposure and cancer.

2. Malcolm Gladwell, "The Paradox of AIDS Politics: Equity for a 'Special' Disease," *Washington Post*, June 23, 1991, p. A10.

3. Some will be inclined to see scientific judgment as inseparable from political motivation.

4. On credit claiming and blame avoidance by politicians, see David R. Mayhew, *Congress: The Electoral Connection* (Yale University Press, 1974); and R. Kent Weaver, "The Politics of Blame Avoidance," *Journal of Public Policy*, vol. 6 (October–December 1986), pp. 371–98.

5. On the significance of contextual goals and the assorted difficulties of reconciling them, see James Q. Wilson, *Bureaucracy: What Government Agencies Do and Why They Do It* (Basic Books, 1989).

6. Dick Thompson, "The AIDS Political Machine," *Time*, January 22, 1990, pp. 24–25. For comments chiding those who would use this term, see June E. Osborn, "Dispelling Myths about the AIDS Epidemic," in Vivian E. Fransen, ed., *Proceedings: AIDS Prevention and Services Workshop—February 15–16, 1990* (Princeton, N.J.: Robert Wood Johnson Foundation Communications Office, June 1990), p. 15. By 1992 some four hundred private foundations were supporting AIDS-related work according to Pamela Sebastian, "Funding a Cause: AIDS Groups Refine Strategies as Many Court Same Donors," *Wall Street Journal*, December 30, 1992, p. 1.

7. Michael Fumento, *The Myth of Heterosexual AIDS* (New Republic/Basic Books, 1990).

8. A well-known premature declaration of triumph over microbial disease is Sir Macfarlane Burnet and David O. White, *Natural History of Infectious*

Disease, 4th ed. (Cambridge University Press, 1972). For a different perspective, see Joshua Lederberg, Robert E. Shope, and Stanley C. Oaks, Jr., eds., *Emerging Infections: Microbial Threats to Health in the United States* (Washington: National Academy Press for the Institute of Medicine, 1992) and the prescient Richard M. Krause, *The Restless Tide: The Persistent Challenge of the Microbial World* (Washington: National Foundation for Infectious Diseases, 1981). Infectious disease has always been viewed as a major problem for developing countries.

9. Daniel M. Fox, "AIDS and the American Health Polity: The History and Prospects of a Crisis of Authority," in Elizabeth Fee and Daniel M. Fox, eds., *AIDS: The Burdens of History* (University of California Press, 1988), pp. 317–20.

10. Belief in HIV as the cause of AIDS is not universal. An alternative but widely challenged view holds that AIDS results from life-style risks (such as use of psychoactive and other drugs) that are immunosuppressive, and that people infected with HIV will not develop AIDS if they avoid these risks. The best-known proponent of this view has been Peter Duesberg, a biologist at the University of California at Berkeley. See, for example, Peter H. Duesberg and Bryan J. Ellison, "Is the AIDS Virus a Science Fiction?" *Policy Review*, no. 53 (Summer 1990), pp. 40–51.

11. Richard E. Neustadt and Harvey V. Fineberg, *The Epidemic That Never Was: Policy-Making and the Swine Flu Scare* (Vintage Books, 1983). A narrative of the Spanish influenza epidemic of 1918–19 is A. A. Hoehling, *The Great Epidemic* (Little, Brown, 1961).

12. Arthur M. Silverstein, *Pure Politics and Impure Science: The Swine Flu Affair* (Johns Hopkins University Press, 1981), p. 98.

13. Peter Applebome, "Mist in Grocery's Produce Section Is Linked to Legionnaires' Disease," *New York Times*, January 11, 1990, pp. A1, D22.

14. Lawrence B. Schonberger and others, "Guillain-Barré Syndrome following Vaccination in the National Influenza Immunization Program, United States, 1976–1977," *American Journal of Epidemiology*, vol. 110 (August 1979), p. 105.

15. Centers for Disease Control, *Morbidity and Mortality Weekly Report*, Atlanta, October 4, 1991, p. 55, table 1. (Hereafter CDC, *MMWR*.)

16. Morton Mintz, *At Any Cost: Corporate Greed, Women, and the Dalkon Shield* (Pantheon, 1985).

17. "Reye Syndrome Surveillance—United States, 1987 and 1988," *MMWR*, May 12, 1989, p. 326.

18. *Infant Formula*, Committee Print, Subcommittee on Oversight and Investigations of the House Committee on Interstate and Foreign Commerce, 96 Cong. 1 sess. (Government Printing Office, 1980); and *Infant Formula: The Present Danger*, Hearing before the Subcommittee on Oversight and Investigations of the House Committee on Energy and Commerce, 97 Cong. 2 sess. (Government Printing Office, 1982).

19. *Tamper-Resistant Packaging for Over-the-Counter Drugs*, Hearing before the Subcommittee on Health and the Environment of the House Committee on Energy and Commerce, 97 Cong. 2 sess. (GPO, 1982). See also Cristine

Russell, "Putting a Lid on Product Tampering," *Washington Post*, May 23, 1986, p. A13.

20. *FDA's Regulation of the Marketing of Unapproved New Drugs: The Case of E-Ferol Vitamin E Aqueous Solution*, Hearing before the Subcommittee on Intergovernmental Relations and Human Resources of the House Committee on Government Operations, 98 Cong. 2 sess. (GPO, 1984).

21. National Institute of Allergy and Infectious Diseases, Office of Communications, *Backgrounder—Lyme Disease* (Rockville, Md.: National Institutes of Health, 1989), pp. 1–2. See also Berton Roueché, "Annals of Medicine: The Foulest and Nastiest Creatures That Be," *New Yorker*, September 12, 1988, pp. 83–89.

22. Malcolm Gladwell, "'72 Diet-Pill Ban Ignored until Recent Deaths," *Washington Post*, September 5, 1990, pp. A1, A15–16.

23. National Institute of Allergy and Infectious Diseases, *Backgrounder—Chronic Fatigue Syndrome* (Rockville, Md., undated), p. 1.

24. Jane Gross, "Women with Breast Implants Split on Need for U.S. Controls," *New York Times*, November 5, 1991, pp. A1, A18.

25. Robert D. McFadden, "A New Tuberculosis Results in 13 Deaths in New York Prisons," *New York Times*, November 16, 1991, pp. 1, 22.

26. Lawrence K. Altman, "Public Health Service Moves to Curb Spread of Drug-Resistant Type of TB," *New York Times*, May 1, 1992, p. A12.

27. CDC, "Update: Multistate Outbreak of *Escherichia coli*," *MMWR*, April 16, 1993, pp. 258–63.

28. CDC, "Outbreak of Acute Illness, Southwestern United States, 1993," *MMWR*, June 11, 1993, p. 421.

29. CDC, "Update: Outbreak of Hantavirus Infection—Southwestern United States, 1993," *MMWR*, June 25, 1993, p. 477.

30. The infectious diseases that are considered in this book are a subset of what public health specialists have called "emerging" diseases, which are those "whose incidence in humans has increased within the past two decades or threatens to increase in the near future." See CDC, *Addressing Emerging Infectious Disease Threats to Health: A Prevention Strategy for the United States* (Atlanta, 1994), p. 1.

31. Norman Zinberg, "Mandatory Testing for Drug Use and AIDS," in Mathea Falco and Warren I. Cikins, eds., *Toward a National Policy on Drug and AIDS Testing* (Brookings, 1989), p. 64.

32. As the Occupational Safety and Health Administration noted in justifying a major new rule on occupational exposure to blood-borne pathogens, including HIV and hepatitis B virus, "A single exposure incident may result in infection and subsequent illness and in some cases, death." See 56 Fed. Reg. 64089 (1991).

33. One indicator of the fear inspired by lethal, uncontrolled infectious disease is the frequency with which popular novelists mine the territory. Three well-known examples are Alistair MacLean, *The Satan Bug* (Fawcett Publications, 1962); Michael Crichton, *The Andromeda Strain* (Knopf, 1969); and Stephen King, *The Stand* (Doubleday, 1978).

34. Paul Brodeur, *The Great Power-Line Cover-up: How the Utilities and the Government Are Trying to Hide the Cancer Hazard Posed by Electromagnetic Fields* (Little, Brown and Company, 1993).

35. For more details on the Alar scare, see Peter Carlson, "The Image Makers," *Washington Post Magazine*, February 11, 1990, pp. 31–32; and Michael Fumento, *Science under Siege: Balancing Technology and the Environment* (William Morrow, 1993), chap. 1. The summer of 1989 also saw a similar episode induced by a government finding of cyanide contamination in a batch of Chilean grapes.

36. On this point, see, for example, Sanford L. Weiner, "Tampons and Toxic Shock Syndrome: Consumer Protection or Public Confusion?" in Harvey M. Sapolsky, *Consuming Fears: The Politics of Product Risks* (Basic Books, 1986), pp. 141–58.

37. Peter M. Sandman, "Hazard versus Outrage in the Public Perception of Risk," in Vincent T. Covello, David B. McCallum, and Maria T. Pavlova, eds., *Effective Risk Communication: The Role and Responsibility of Government and Nongovernment Organizations* (Plenum, 1989), pp. 45–49.

38. Elizabeth Fee, *Disease and Discovery: A History of the Johns Hopkins School of Hygiene and Public Health, 1916–1939* (Johns Hopkins University Press, 1987), p. 10. See also John Duffy, *The Sanitarians: A History of American Public Health* (University of Illinois Press, 1990).

39. Charles L. Schultze, *The Public Use of Private Interest* (Brookings, 1977), pp. 70–72.

40. Examples include Allan M. Brandt, *No Magic Bullet: A Social History of Venereal Disease in the United States since 1880* (Oxford University Press, 1987); Mary Douglas and Aaron Wildavsky, *Risk and Culture: An Essay on the Selection of Technological and Environmental Dangers* (University of California Press, 1982); and Branden B. Johnson and Vincent T. Covello, eds., *The Social and Cultural Construction of Risk: Essays on Risk Selection and Perception* (Dordrecht, Holland: D. Reidel, 1987).

41. Charles E. Rosenberg, *The Cholera Years: The United States in 1832, 1849, and 1866* (University of Chicago Press, 1962); and J. H. Powell, *Bring Out Your Dead: The Great Plague of Yellow Fever in Philadelphia in 1793* (University of Pennsylvania Press, 1949).

42. Daniel Kahneman and Amos Tversky, "The Psychology of Preferences," *Scientific American*, vol. 246 (January 1982), pp. 160–73; and Kahneman and Tversky, "Choices, Values, and Frames," *American Psychologist*, vol. 39 (April 1984), pp. 341–50.

43. Aaron Wildavsky, *Searching for Safety* (Transaction Books, 1988). This volume contains the major statement of Wildavsky's normative argument on health and safety risks. Elsewhere he has also offered an empirical argument, asking "Why do we fear the things we do?" For examples of the cultural approach he employs to answer this latter question, see Douglas and Wildavsky, *Risk and Culture*; and Aaron Wildavsky and Karl Dake, "Theories of Risk Perception: Who Fears What and Why?" *Daedalus*, vol. 119 (Fall 1990), pp. 41–60.

44. Lawrence K. Altman, "Rare Cancer Seen in 41 Homosexuals," *New York Times*, July 3, 1981, p. A20.

45. Albert R. Jonsen and Jeff Stryker, eds., *The Social Impact of AIDS in the United States* (Washington: National Academy Press, 1993), p. 30.

46. See, for example, the statement by Mel Rosen of the Gay Men's Health Crisis in *Federal Response to AIDS*, Hearing before the Subcommittee on Intergovernmental Relations and Human Resources of the House Committee on Government Operations, 98 Cong. 1 sess. (GPO, 1983), p. 189. See also Charles Perrow and Mauro F. Guillén, *The AIDS Disaster: The Failure of Organizations in New York and the Nation* (Yale University Press, 1990), p. 46.

Chapter Two

1. See C. Arden Miller and Merry-K. Moos, *Local Health Departments: Fifteen Case Studies* (Washington: American Public Health Association, 1981); National Association of County Health Officials, *National Profile of Local Health Departments: An Overview of the Nation's Local Public Health System* (Washington: National Association of County Health Officials, 1990); Public Health Practice Program Office, *Profile of State and Territorial Public Health Systems: United States, 1990* (Atlanta, Ga.: Centers for Disease Control, December 1991).

2. Committee for the Study of the Future of Public Health, Institute of Medicine, *The Future of Public Health* (Washington: National Academy Press, 1988), p. 3. On this point, see also Edward F. Lawlor, "When a Possible Job Becomes Impossible: Politics, Public Health, and the Management of the AIDS Epidemic," in Erwin C. Hargrove and John C. Glidewell, eds., *Impossible Jobs in Public Management* (University Press of Kansas, 1990), p. 153.

3. Centers for Disease Control, Division of STD/HIV Prevention, *Annual Report—1992*, pp. 79–80.

4. On this epidemic, see Marcia Goldoft and John Kobayashi, "Scientific Work and Epidemiologic Vigilance Quickly Halt E. Coli Epidemic," *Washington Public Health*, vol. 11 (Fall 1993), pp. 1–3.

5. Lawlor, "When a Possible Job Becomes Impossible," p. 154.

6. Ibid., p. 155.

7. Obviously the politician personally victimized by a hazard may manifest public concern about it regardless of the constituency he or she formally represents. Representatives Berkley Bedell, Democrat of Iowa, and Kenneth J. Gray, Democrat of Illinois, were forced into early retirement from Congress as a result of contracting Lyme disease. Though neither represented an area particularly associated with the disease both later lobbied their former colleagues to sponsor legislation supporting Lyme disease research and education. See draft letter to members of Congress dated April 7, 1989, by Berkley Bedell and Kenneth J. Gray in support of the Comprehensive Lyme Disease Act of 1989.

8. Christopher H. Foreman, Jr., *Signals from the Hill: Congressional Oversight and the Challenge of Social Regulation* (Yale University Press, 1988).

9. See, for example, *Risking America's Health and Safety: George Bush and the Task Force on Regulatory Relief* (Washington: Public Citizen, October 1988), pp. 8–9, 14–15.

10. Health threats accorded public prominence and increased research funding partly as a result of this kind of mobilization include sudden infant death syndrome (SIDS) and Alzheimer's disease. See Abraham B. Bergman, *The "Discovery" of Sudden Infant Death Syndrome: Lessons in the Practice of Political Medicine* (Praeger, 1986); and Patrick Fox, "From Senility to Alzheimer's Disease: The Rise of the Alzheimer's Disease Movement," *Milbank Quarterly*, vol. 67, no. 1 (1989), pp. 58–102.

11. Michael Pertschuk, *Giant Killers* (W. W. Norton, 1986), pp. 51–52.

12. Robert M. Wachter, "AIDS, Activism, and the Politics of Health," *New England Journal of Medicine*, January 9, 1992, pp. 128–33.

13. David R. Mayhew, *Congress: The Electoral Connection* (Yale University Press, 1974).

14. Terry M. Moe, "The Politics of Bureaucratic Structure," in John E. Chubb and Paul E. Peterson, eds., *Can the Government Govern?* (Brookings, 1989), p. 269.

15. Donald L. Horowitz, *The Courts and Social Policy* (Brookings, 1977).

16. A useful overview of the various forces at work in media treatment of the scientific and technological aspects of risk is a background paper by Dorothy Nelkin, *Science in the Streets: Report of the Twentieth Century Fund Task Force on the Communication of Scientific Risk* (Priority Press, 1984).

17. Stephen Klaidman, *Health in the Headlines: The Stories behind the Stories* (Oxford University Press, 1991), p. 9.

18. Lisa Leff, "U-Md. Takes Meningitis Precautions: 100 Get Antibiotics after Student Dies," *Washington Post*, April 10, 1992, p. A24.

19. Anthony Schmitz, "Food News Blues," *In Health*, vol. 5 (November 1991), pp. 40–45.

20. Dorothy Nelkin, *Selling Science: How the Press Covers Science and Technology* (W. H. Freeman, 1987), p. 77.

21. An example is the Pulitzer Prize-winning reporting on the U.S. blood industry by Gilbert M. Gaul of the Philadelphia Inquirer. His work is reprinted in Kendall J. Wills, ed., *The Pulitzer Prizes—1990* (Simon and Schuster, 1990), pp. 31–109.

22. See Randy Shilts, *And the Band Played On: Politics, People, and the AIDS Epidemic* (St. Martin's Press, 1987); and James Kinsella, *Covering the Plague: AIDS and the American Media* (Rutgers University Press, 1989).

23. Doris A. Graber, *Mass Media and American Politics*, 4th ed. (Washington: Congressional Quarterly Press, 1993), chap. 3. On the role of such factors in reporting on science and technology particularly, see Nelkin, *Selling Science*. See also Edward Jay Epstein, *News from Nowhere: Television and the News* (Random House, 1973).

24. Mary Harvey, Ralph I. Horwitz, and Alvan R. Feinstein, "Toxic Shock and Tampons: Evaluation of the Epidemiologic Evidence," *Journal of the American Medical Association*, August 20, 1982, pp. 840–46.

25. For example, research into the relationship between reporters and scientific experts discloses a strong journalistic predilection in favor of experts skeptical of both nuclear energy and intelligence testing—a skepticism sharply at odds with the majority of expert opinion in both fields. See Stanley Rothman,

"Journalists, Broadcasters, Scientific Experts and Public Opinion," *Minerva*, vol. 28 (Summer 1990), pp. 117–33.

26. Robert D. McFadden, "Child in Tampering Scare Had Been Ill," *New York Times*, October 20, 1991, p. 25; and Calvin Sims, "Girl Not Killed by Baby Food, Examiner Says," *New York Times*, November 16, 1991, p. 22.

27. Lawrence K. Altman, "Deadly Strain of Tuberculosis Is Spreading Fast, U.S. Finds," *New York Times*, January 24, 1992, pp. A1, B6; and Altman, "For Most, Risk of Contracting Tuberculosis Is Seen as Small," *New York Times*, January 25, 1992, pp. 1, 9.

28. Fitzhugh Mullan, *Plagues and Politics: The Story of the United States Public Health Service* (Basic Books, 1989), p. 14.

29. Charles E. Rosenberg, *The Cholera Years: The United States in 1832, 1849, and 1866* (University of Chicago Press, 1987), pp. 47–53. See also Charles Warren, *Odd Byways in American History* (Harvard University Press, 1942), chap. 12.

30. National Institutes of Health, *NIH Data Book—1993* (Bethesda, Md., 1993), p. ii.

31. Ibid., pp. 10, 20.

32. On the political environment of the NIH, see Stephen P. Strickland, *Politics, Science and Dread Disease: A Short History of United States Medical Research Policy* (Harvard University Press, 1972); Natalie Davis Spingarn, *Heartbeat: The Politics of Health Research* (Washington and New York: Robert B. Luce, 1976); and Rufus E. Miles, Jr., *The Department of Health, Education, and Welfare* (Praeger, 1974), pp. 168–90. Congress has also enacted legislation calling for special efforts within or among institutes for such ailments as sickle cell anemia and sudden infant death syndrome. See Thomas J. Kennedy, Jr., and Ivan L. Bennett, Jr., "The Planning of Research: The Role of the Federal Government," in Henry Wechsler, Ronald W. Lamont-Havers, and George F. Cahill, Jr., *The Social Context of Medical Research* (Ballinger, 1981), p. 47.

33. David Vogel, "AIDS and the Politics of Drug Lag," *Public Interest*, no. 96 (Summer 1989), pp. 73–85.

34. The implications of this for legislative oversight of FDA are discussed in Foreman, *Signals from the Hill*, pp. 45–55, and passim.

35. Marian Burros, "The Saga of a Food Regulation: After 25 Years, Still No Decision," *New York Times*, February 13, 1985, pp. C1, C8.

36. During an interview, one former NIH institute director highlighted the difference in institutional culture between the NIH and the CDC by observing that while his own organization included many members of the prestigious National Academy of Sciences, the CDC had none.

37. See generally Elizabeth W. Etheridge, *Sentinel for Health: A History of the Centers for Disease Control* (University of California Press, 1992).

38. On these difficulties, see Etheridge, *Sentinel for Health*, p. 58.

39. On the origins of the surgeon general, see Mullan, *Plagues and Politics*, chap. 1.

40. On the origins of the reorganization that abolished the surgeon general's authority to run the PHS, see Mullan, *Plagues and Politics*, pp. 154, 158, 162.

41. Mullan, *Plagues and Politics*, p. 173.

42. An exception in this regard was the 1969 effort by HEW Secretary Robert Finch to persuade President Richard Nixon to appoint John H. Knowles, head of Boston's Massachusetts General Hospital, assistant secretary for health. Vigorous opposition by the American Medical Association and by a key congressional ally, Senate Minority Leader Everett McKinley Dirksen, Republican of Illinois), resulted in an unsuccessful five-month struggle by Finch to win the appointment for Knowles. See E. W. Kenworthy, "Finch Drops Fight to Give Knowles Top Health Post," *New York Times*, June 28, 1969, pp. 1, 16.

43. See Shilts, *And the Band Played On*, chap. 29.

44. Joseph A. Califano, Jr., *Governing America: An Insider's Report from the White House and the Cabinet* (Simon and Schuster, 1981), pp. 173–74.

45. John H. Trattner, *The Prune Book: The 100 Toughest Management and Policy-Making Jobs in Washington* (Lanham, Md.: Madison Books, 1988), pp. 274–78.

Chapter Three

1. Centers for Disease Control, "Guidelines for Investigating Clusters of Health Events," *Morbidity and Mortality Weekly Report*, Atlanta, July 27, 1990, p. 1. (Hereafter CDC, *MMWR*.)

2. A passive system of surveillance is so designated because "no action is taken unless completed reports are received by the public health agency." An active system "involves an ongoing search for cases." Passive systems are cheaper but generate less complete reporting than active systems. Gregory R. Istre, "Disease Surveillance at the State and Local Levels," in William Halperin, Edward L. Baker, Jr., and Richard R. Monson, *Public Health Surveillance* (Van Nostrand Reinhold, 1992), pp. 46–48.

3. CDC, "Guidelines for Evaluating Surveillance Systems," *MMWR*, supplement, May 6, 1988, p. 1. The following discussion of surveillance draws generally on this document.

4. Abraham M. Lilienfeld and David E. Lilienfeld, *Foundations of Epidemiology*, 2d ed. (Oxford University Press, 1980), chap. 8.

5. On the nature of postmarketing surveillance, see Hugh H. Tilson, "Pharmacosurveillance: Public Health Monitoring of Medication," in Halperin, Baker, Jr., and Monson, *Public Health Surveillance*, pp. 206–29.

6. Remarks of FDA Commissioner David A. Kessler to Medwatch meeting dated June 3, 1993.

7. One commentator reported that the FDA developed a significant program of adverse experience monitoring only in the 1950s in response to reports of aplastic anemia in association with use of the antibiotic chloramphenicol. See Gerald A. Faich, "Special Report: Adverse Drug Reaction Monitoring," *New England Journal of Medicine*, June 12, 1986, p. 1589. See also Geoffrey R. Venning, "Identification of Adverse Reactions to New Drugs. II—How Were 18 Important Adverse Reactions Discovered and with What Delays?" *British Medical Journal*, January 22, 1983, p. 291.

8. William H. Foege, "Uses of Epidemiology in the Development of Health Policy," *Public Health Reports*, vol. 99 (May–June 1984), p. 234. The diverse

earlier efforts are discussed in Stephen B. Thacker and Ruth L. Berkelman, "History of Public Health Surveillance," in Halperin, Baker, and Monson, *Public Health Surveillance*, pp. 1–15.

9. On the background of NETSS, see Philip L. Graitcer and Anthony H. Burton, "The Epidemiologic Surveillance Project: A Computer-Based System for Disease Surveillance," *American Journal of Preventive Medicine*, vol. 3, no. 3 (1987), pp. 123–27.

10. Istre, "Disease Surveillance," p. 46.

11. General Accounting Office, *Federal Regulation of Medical Devices— Problems Still to be Overcome*, GAO/HRD-83-53 (Washington, September 1983), *Medical Devices: Early Warning of Problems Is Hampered by Severe Underreporting*, GAO/PEMB-87-1 (Washington, December 1986), *Seafood Safety: Seriousness of Problems and Efforts to Protect Consumers*, GAO/RCED-88-135 (Washington, August 1988), *At Risk*, GAO/T-PEMD-90-2 (Washington, November 1989), and *Medical Devices: Underreporting of Serious Problems with Home Apnea Monitor*, GAO/PEMD-90-17 (Washington, May 1990).

12. Istre, "Disease Surveillance," pp. 43–44.

13. CDC, "Surveillance of Elevated Blood Lead Levels among Adults— United States, 1992," *MMWR*, May 1, 1992, p. 285.

14. "Lyme Disease Surveillance—United States, 1989-1990," *MMWR*, June 28, 1991, pp. 417–21.

15. Lawrence K. Altman, "Communicable Disease Masked behind Doctors' Erratic Reporting," *New York Times*, July 10, 1990, p. C3.

16. Stephen B. Thacker and Ruth L. Berkelman, "History of Public Health Surveillance," in Halperin, Baker, Jr., and Monson, *Public Health Surveillance*, p. 4.

17. Altman, "Communicable Diseases."

18. James M. Hughes and Morris E. Potter, "Scombroid-Fish Poisoning: From Pathogenesis to Prevention," *New England Journal of Medicine*, March 14, 1991, p. 766.

19. By the fall of 1992, for example, government officials were concerned that as many as half of the cases that would meet the CDC surveillance criteria of L-tryptophan-related eosinophilia-myalgia syndrome had gone unreported. See Food and Drug Administration, "Dear Colleague" letter on eosinophilia-myalgia syndrome and L-tryptophan dated September 3, 1992, p. 2.

20. June E. Osborn, "Dispelling Myths about the AIDS Epidemic," in Vivian E. Fransen, *Proceedings: AIDS Prevention and Services Workshop—February 15–16, 1990* (Princeton, N.J.: Robert Wood Johnson Foundation Communication Office, June 1990), p. 18.

21. On this last point, see, for example, Joann M. Schulte, Frederick A. Martich, and George P. Schmid, "Chancroid in the United States, 1981–1990: Evidence for Underreporting of Cases," *MMWR*, May 29, 1992, pp. 57–61.

22. An exception is Joshua Lederberg, Robert E. Shope, and Stanley C. Oaks, Jr., *Emerging Infections: Microbial Threats to Health in the United States* (Washington: National Academy Press, 1992), chap. 3.

23. On this point, see CDC, "Guidelines for Evaluating Surveillance Systems," *MMWR*, p. 9.

24. Jack W. Hopkins, *The Eradication of Smallpox: Organizational Learning and Innovation in International Health* (Westview Press, 1989). See also Thacker and Berkelman, "History," p. 5.

25. On the uses of case-control studies and the ways they differ from the far more resource-intensive prospective studies that rely on mass sampling, see Abraham M. Lilienfeld and David E. Lilienfeld, *Foundations of Epidemiology*, 2d ed. (Oxford University Press, 1980), chaps. 8, 9.

26. Mary Harvey, Ralph I. Horwitz, and Alvan R. Feinstein, "Toxic Shock and Tampons: Evaluation of the Epidemiologic Evidence," *Journal of the American Medical Association*, August 20, 1982, pp. 840–46. See also Alvan R. Feinstein, "Scientific Standards in Epidemiologic Studies of the Menace of Daily Life," *Science*, December 2, 1988, pp. 1257–63.

27. Marcia Barinaga, "Furor at Lyme Conference," *Science*, June 5, 1992, pp. 1384–85.

28. Malcolm Gladwell, "There May Be Nothing Unsafe in the Numbers about Halcion," *Washington Post*, June 15, 1992, p. A3.

29. On the problem of bias in drug reaction reporting, see R. M. Sachs and E. A. Bortnichak, "An Evaluation of Spontaneous Adverse Drug Reaction Monitoring Systems," *American Journal of Medicine*, November 28, 1986, pp. 49–55.

30. Malcolm Gladwell, "Officials Respond Cautiously to Reports of Mysterious AIDS-Like Disease," *Washington Post*, July 22, 1992, p. A4.

31. Lawrence K. Altman, "C.D.C. Is Embarrassed by Its Tardy Response to AIDS-Like Illness," *New York Times*, July 28, 1992, p. C3.

32. Morton Mintz, *At Any Cost: Corporate Greed, Women, and the Dalkon Shield* (Pantheon Books, 1985).

33. Gina Kolata, "Manufacturer of Faulty Heart Valve Barred Data on Dangers, F.D.A. Says," *New York Times*, March 21, 1992, p. 50. In 1994, FDA concluded that the Upjohn Company might have hidden unfavorable data on Halcion. See John Schwartz, "Halcion's Effects Hidden, FDA Investigators Claim," *Washington Post*, April 26, 1994, p. A3.

34. Cristine Russell, "Centers for Disease Control: 40 Years of Demystifying Illness," *Washington Post*, September 4, 1986, p. A15.

35. A related factor may be that the medical profession has long employed published descriptions of unusual patients as a way of alerting members to new developments. The correspondence section of virtually any issue of the *New England Journal of Medicine* offers examples.

36. Stephen S. Morse, "Regulating Viral Traffic," *Issues in Science and Technology*, vol. 7 (Fall 1990), pp. 81–84.

37. Mysterious outbreaks of respiratory disease in a Washington, D.C., hospital in 1965 and in Pontiac, Michigan, in 1969 would later be attributed to Legionnaires' disease. See *Legionnaires' Disease*, 1977, Hearings before the Subcommittee on Health and Scientific Research of the Senate Committee on

Human Resources, 95 Cong. 1 sess. (Washington: Government Printing Office, 1978), esp. pp. 5, 7–8.

38. Christine Gorman, "Strange Trip Back to the Future," *Time*, November 9, 1987, p. 83; and Matt Clark, "A New Clue in the AIDS Mystery," *Newsweek*, November 9, 1987, p. 62.

39. Lawrence K. Altman, "Puzzle of Sailor's Death Solved after 31 Years: The Answer Is AIDS," *New York Times*, July 24, 1990, p. C3.

40. Randy Shilts, *And the Band Played On: Politics, People, and the AIDS Epidemic* (St. Martin's Press, 1987), p. 49.

41. Ibid., pp. 42–43, 56. An earlier account of the discovery of AIDS is contained in Gerald Astor, *The Disease Detectives: Medical Mysteries and the People Who Solved Them* (New American Library, 1983), pp. 53–63.

42. Shilts, *And the Band Played On*, pp. 64–65. As Shilts reported, the CDC also got wind of the epidemic by a different route, via a staff technician's suspicions about an unusual cluster of orders for pentamidine, a drug used to fight *Pneumocystis carinii* pneumonia. See pp. 54, 61, and 66.

43. Ibid., pp. 68–69; and CDC, "*Pneumocystis* Pneumonia—Los Angeles," *MMWR*, June 5, 1981, pp. 250–52.

44. Gerald M. Oppenheimer, "In the Eye of the Storm: The Epidemiological Construction of AIDS," in Elizabeth Fee and Daniel M. Fox, eds., *AIDS: The Burdens of History* (University of California Press, 1988), p. 271.

45. One commentator has suggested that CDC policymakers expected considerable media interest and were mystified by its failure to materialize. See James Kinsella, *Covering the Plague: AIDS and the American Media* (Rutgers University Press, 1989), pp. 8–11.

46. This discussion of toxic shock syndrome relies upon Sanford L. Weiner, "Tampons and Toxic Shock Syndrome: Consumer Protection or Public Confusion?" in Harvey M. Sapolsky, ed., *Consuming Fears: The Politics of Product Risks* (Basic Books, 1986), pp. 141–58; Maria E. Donawa, George R. Schmid, and Michael T. Osterholm, "Toxic Shock Syndrome: Chronology of State and Federal Epidemiologic Studies and Regulatory Decision-Making," *Public Health Reports*, vol. 99 (July-August 1984), pp. 342–50; and Mary Harvey, Ralph I. Horwitz, and Alvan R. Feinstein, "Toxic Shock and Tampons," *Journal of the American Medical Association*, pp. 840–46. Some have hypothesized that toxic shock syndrome may have played a role in the oldest recorded high mortality epidemic, the so-called plague of Athens that broke out in Attica, Greece, in 430 B.C. See Alexander D. Langmuir and others, "The Thucydides Syndrome: A New Hypothesis for the Cause of the Plague of Athens," *New England Journal of Medicine*, October 17, 1985, pp. 1027–30.

47. Weiner, "Tampons and Toxic Shock," p. 142.

48. Ibid., p. 143.

49. J. Donald Millar and June E. Osborn, "Precursors of the Scientific Decision-Making Process Leading to the 1976 National Immunization Campaign," in June E. Osborn, ed., *Influenza in America, 1918-1976: History, Science, and Politics* (Prodist, 1977), p. 24. See more generally the appendix titled "Swine

Flu Chronology" in Richard E. Neustadt and Harvey V. Fineberg, *The Epidemic That Never Was: Policy-Making and the Swine Flu Scare* (Vintage, 1983), pp. 164–69.

50. Barton J. Bernstein, "The Swine Flu Vaccination Campaign of 1976: Politics, Science, and the Public," *Congress and the Presidency*, vol. 10 (Spring 1983), p. 95.

51. I have adapted the material in these paragraphs from Joel Lang, "Catching the Bug: How Scientists Found the Cause of Lyme Disease and Why We're Not Out of the Woods Yet," *Connecticut Medicine*, vol. 53 (June 1989), pp. 357–64.

52. Robert A. Aronowitz, "Lyme Disease: The Social Construction of a New Disease and Its Social Consequences," *Milbank Quarterly*, vol. 69, no. 1 (1991), p. 93.

53. This account is taken from *Infant Formula: Our Children Need Better Protection*, Committee Print 96-IFC 42, Subcommittee on Oversight and Investigation of the House Committee on Interstate and Foreign Commerce, 96 Cong. 2 sess. (GPO, 1980).

54. Ibid., p. 5.

55. This and later discussions of L-tryptophan were drawn from a Pulitzer Prize-winning series of seven newspaper articles by Tamar Stieber of the *Albuquerque Journal*. The articles have been reprinted in Kendall J. Wills, ed., *The Pulitzer Prizes: 1990* (Simon and Schuster, 1990), pp. 451–80. See p. 457 for quotation.

56. Ibid., p. 459. See also Benedict Carey, "Bitter Pill," *In Health*, vol. 5 (January–February 1991), p. 76.

57. This material is adapted from Geoffrey Cowley, "Chronic Fatigue Syndrome: A Modern Medical Mystery," *Newsweek*, November 12, 1990, pp. 62–70.

58. Ibid., p. 64. Emphasis in original.

59. In recent years, the CDC has received fewer than twenty annual reports of such diseases as plague, diptheria, and cholera. Even allowing for underreporting, such data suggest problems of a manageable scale. See CDC, "Summary of Notifiable Diseases, United States, 1991," *MMWR*, October 2, 1992, p. 57.

60. Ruth L. Berkelman, James W. Buehler, and Timothy J. Dondero, Jr., "Surveillance of Acquired Immunodeficiency Syndrome (AIDS)," in Halperin, Baker, and Monson, *Public Health Surveillance*, p. 109.

61. The EIS, established after World War II, offers epidemiologic training to selected public health professionals who give two years of EIS service in return. That service often includes assignment to a state or local health authority, sometimes to help monitor and combat disease outbreaks. EIS officers have been intimately involved in several of the episodes discussed in this book. See, generally, Alexander D. Langmuir, "The Epidemic Intelligence Service of the Centers for Disease Control," *Public Health Reports*, vol. 95 (September–October 1980), pp. 470–77.

62. Richard A. Goodman and others, "Epidemiologic Field Investigations by the Centers for Disease Control and the Epidemic Intelligence Service, 1946–87," *Public Health Reports*, vol. 105 (November–December 1990), pp. 604–10 (quotation on p. 605).

63. *Legionnaires' Disease*, 1977, Hearings, p. 85.

64. Berton Roueché, *The Medical Detectives* (Pocket Books, 1980), chap. 6.

65. Goodman and others, "Epidemiologic Field Investigations," p. 605.

66. Generally speaking, this is one of the main differences between surveillance and an epidemiologic study. The ongoing nature of surveillance means that it must be kept fairly simple and unburdensome for participants, unlike the more demanding detailed studies examining alternative risk factors and explanatory hypotheses. And because a key aim of nationally sponsored surveillance is to provide data that state and local officials can promptly use, the simplicity of data dissemination is important as well.

67. On the last of these examples, see Bruce Lambert, "4 Cases Found of Rare Strain of AIDS Virus," *New York Times*, June 27, 1989, pp. B1, B4.

68. Dixie E. Snider, Jr., Louis Salinas, and Gloria D. Kelly, "Tuberculosis: An Increasing Problem among Minorities in the United States," *Public Health Reports*, vol. 104 (November–December 1989), p. 647.

69. See the comments of CDC Director David J. Sencer in *Legionnaires' Disease*, Hearings before the Subcommittee on Consumer Protection and Finance of the House Committee on Interstate and Foreign Commerce, 94 Cong. 2 sess. (GPO, 1977), p. 110.

70. See, for example, Larry Kramer, *Reports from the holocaust: The Making of an AIDS Activist* (St. Martin's Press, 1989), p. 26.

71. A colorful and detailed recounting is Gordon Thomas and Max Morgan-Witts, *Anatomy of an Epidemic* (Doubleday, 1982).

72. See the testimony of Edward T. Hoak in *Legionnaires' Disease*, 1977, Hearings, pp. 156–59.

73. Ibid., p. 99.

74. On this final point, see the discussion in Shilts, *And the Band Played On*, p. 19.

75. I draw here upon Kinsella, *Covering the Plague*, chaps. 4, 5.

76. CDC, *HIV/AIDS Surveillance Report* (Atlanta, December 1989), p. 11. See also Kinsella, *Covering the Plague*, pp. 18–19; and CDC, "Possible Transfusion-Associated Acquired Immune Deficiency Syndrome (AIDS)—California," *MMWR*, December 10, 1982, pp. 652–54.

77. John Z. Sullivan-Bolyai and Lawrence Corey, "Epidemiology of Reye Syndrome," *Epidemiologic Reviews*, vol. 3 (1981), p. 2.

78. This quotation from the *MMWR* appears in Oppenheimer, "In the Eye of the Storm," p. 272.

79. Ibid.

80. See *Reye's Syndrome*, Hearings before the Subcommittee on Natural Resources, Agriculture Research and Environment before the House Committee on Science and Technology, 97 Cong. 2 sess. (GPO, 1982).

81. Lawrence K. Altman, "Chronic Fatigue Syndrome Finally Gets Some Respect," *New York Times*, December 4, 1990, pp. C1, C14.

82. Mitchell Zoler, "Taking the Syndrome Seriously: Chronic Fatigue," *Medical World News*, December 12, 1988, p. 33.

83. Gary P. Holmes and others, "Chronic Fatigue Syndrome: A Working Case Definition," *Annals of Internal Medicine*, vol. 108 (1988), pp. 387–89.

84. In a "Dear Colleague" letter on the L-tryptophan-related eosinophilia-myalgia syndrome dated September 3, 1992 (p. 2), the FDA referred to a CDC estimate that "some 3,000 individuals who have consumed LT [L-tryptophan] are now exhibiting symptoms compatible with EMS, but do not fully meet the surveillance criteria for EMS." The letter went on to note that "CDC emphasizes that the published case-definition for surveillance was not intended to be used as diagnostic criteria, and that each case should be judged on its own merits."

85. One authoritative source noted that "fairly early in the [HIV] epidemic, it became apparent that many infected individuals who suffered from clinical symptoms and laboratory abnormalities signaling the presence of HIV infection did not meet the CDC criteria for the disease." Nonetheless, "some of them seemed to develop AIDS at a rapid pace." These individuals were said to have ARC. Institute of Medicine, *Confronting AIDS: Update 1988* (Washington: National Academy Press, 1988), pp. 36–37.

86. The AIDS case definition controversy is comprehensively reviewed in Office of Technology Assessment, *The CDC's Case Definition of AIDS: Implications of the Proposed Revisions* (GPO, August 1992).

87. Mireya Navarro, "Dated AIDS Definition Keeps Benefits from Many Patients," *New York Times*, July 8, 1991, pp. A1, B5.

88. Philip J. Hilts, "AIDS Definition Excludes Women, Congress Is Told," *New York Times*, June 7, 1991, p. A19.

89. Robert Pear, "U.S. Will Relax Disability Rules in H.I.V. Cases," *New York Times*, June 29, 1993, p. A1.

90. Office of Technology Assessment, *CDC's Case Definition of AIDS*, p. 9.

91. Ibid.

92. Mireya Navarro, "More Cases, Costs, and Fears under Wider AIDS Umbrella," *New York Times*, October 29, 1992, pp. A1, B2.

93. General Accounting Office, *AIDS: CDC's Investigation of HIV Transmissions by a Dentist*, GAO/PEMD-92-31 (Washington, September 1992).

94. House of Representatives, Committee on Government Operations, *The FDA's Regulation of Silicone Breast Implants*, Committee Print, Subcommittee on Human Resources and Intergovernmental Relations of the House Committee on Governmental Operations, 102 Cong. 2 sess. (GPO, 1993), esp. pp. 13–15, 22-24.

95. This description appears in a fact sheet, "Survey of Health and AIDS Risk Prevalence," by the Consortium of Social Science Associations (COSSA), Washington, D.C., which strongly supported the survey.

96. Letter to OMB Director Richard G. Darman from Senator Paul Simon, Democrat of Illinois, and others dated March 8, 1989. See also letter from Representative Bill Green, Republican of New York, and others to HHS Secretary Louis W. Sullivan dated June 1, 1989.

97. *Departments of Labor, Health and Human Services, and Education and Related Agencies Appropriation Bill, 1991*, S. Rept. 101-516, 101 Cong. 2 sess. (GPO, 1990), p. 215.

98. *Department of Labor, Health and Human Services, and Education, and Related Agencies Appropriations Bill,* 1991, H. Rept. 101-591, 101 Cong. 2 sess. (GPO, 1990), p. 71.

99. "Dear Colleague" letter from Rep. William E. Dannemeyer, Republican of California, April 11, 1989.

100. Letter from OMB Director Richard G. Darman to HHS Secretary Louis W. Sullivan, April 6, 1989.

101. *HHS News* (press release), April 7, 1989.

102. See National Institutes of Health Revitalization Act of 1993, Public Law 103-43 (107 Stat. 122).

103. Michael Specter, "What's America Doing in Bed?" *Washington Post,* February 25, 1990, pp. B1, B2.

104. Ronald Bayer, *Private Acts, Social Consequences: AIDS and the Politics of Public Health* (Free Press, 1989), p. 117.

105. James K. Todd, "Toxic Shock Syndrome—Scientific Uncertainty and the Public Media," *Pediatrics,* vol. 67 (June 1981), p. 922.

106. Harris L. Coulter and Barbara Loe Fisher, *A Shot in the Dark: Why the P in the DPT Vaccination May Be Hazardous to Your Child's Health* (Avery Publishing Group, 1991).

107. Britain's National Childhood Encephalopathy Study, a large three-year case-control study released in 1981, indicated "the attributable risk . . . of serious neurologic illness in the 7 days following pertussis vaccination [is] 1 in 110,000 immunizations, and that of persistent neurologic damage after 1 year is estimated to be 1 in 310,000 immunizations (with wide confidence limits in both cases)." See Christopher P. Howson, Cynthia J. Howe, and Harvey V. Fineberg, eds., *Adverse Effects of Pertussis and Rubella Vaccines* (Washington: National Academy Press for the Institute of Medicine, 1991), p. 323, appendix B. See also Alan R. Hinman and Jeffrey P. Koplan, "Pertussis and Pertussis Vaccine: Reanalysis of Benefits, Risks, and Costs," *Journal of the American Medical Association,* June 15, 1984, pp. 3109–13.

108. For another example of this phenomenon, see House of Representatives, Committee on Government Operations, *Oversight Review of CDC's Agent Orange Study,* Hearing before the Subcommittee on Human Resources and Intergovernmental Relations of the House Committee on Government Operations, 101 Cong. 1 sess. (GPO, 1990); and the subsequent report, *The Agent Orange Coverup: A Case of Flawed Science and Political Manipulation,* H. Rept. 101-672, 101 Cong. 2 sess. (GPO, 1990).

109. *Legionnaires' Disease,* 1977, Hearings, pp. 16–22.

110. Ibid., p. 22.

111. Astor, *The Disease Detectives,* pp. 25–26. See also Elizabeth W. Etheridge, *Sentinel for Health: A History of the Centers for Disease Control* (University of California Press, 1992), chap. 18.

112. *Legionnaires' Disease,* Hearings before the Subcommittee on Consumer Protection and Finance of the House Committee on Interstate and Foreign Commerce, 94 Cong. 2 sess. (GPO, 1977).

113. See, for example, Mirko D. Grmek, *History of AIDS: Emergence and Origin of a Modern Pandemic* (Princeton University Press, 1990), pp. 15, 106.

114. Thomas and Morgan-Witts, *Anatomy of an Epidemic*, pp. 363–73.

115. Joseph A. Califano, Jr., *Governing America: An Insider's Report from the White House and the Cabinet* (Simon and Schuster, 1981), p. 174.

116. Diana Jean Schemo, "Prolonged Lyme Treatments Posing Risks, Experts Warn," *New York Times*, January 4, 1994, pp. A1, B5.

117. Joseph Palca, "On the Track of an Elusive Disease," *Science*, December 20, 1991, pp. 1726–28. Section 902 of Public Law 103-43, the 1993 NIH Revitalization Act, provides explicitly for an NIH infrastructure for the disease.

118. Speculation first arose that the popularity of nitrate inhalants (or "poppers") among some homosexuals might be linked to the spread of the mysterious ailment.

119. *Kaposi's Sarcoma and Related Opportunistic Infections*, Hearing before the Subcommittee on Health and the Environment of the House Committee on Energy and Commerce, 97 Cong. 2 sess. (GPO, 1982).

120. Sandra Panem, *The AIDS Bureaucracy* (Harvard University Press, 1988), pp. 32–35.

121. Janet S. St. Lawrence, Harold V. Hood, Ted Brasfield, and Jeffrey A. Kelly, "Differences in Gay Men's AIDS Risk Knowledge and Behavior Patterns in High and Low AIDS Prevalence Cities," *Public Health Reports*, vol. 104 (July–August 1989), pp. 391–95. See also David Gelman, "The Young and the Reckless," *Newsweek*, January 11, 1993, pp. 60–61.

122. See, for example, the drastically different perspectives on the growth of the epidemic in Dennis J. Bregman and Alexander D. Langmuir, "Farr's Law Applied to AIDS Projections," *Journal of the American Medical Association*, March 16, 1990, pp. 1538–40, and Renslow Sherer, "AIDS Policy into the 1990s," *Journal of the American Medical Association*, April 11, 1990, pp. 1972–74. See also Michael Fumento, *The Myth of Heterosexual AIDS* (New Republic Books/Basic Books, 1990).

123. Richard E. Neustadt and Harvey V. Fineberg, *The Epidemic That Never Was: Policy-Making and the Swine Flu Scare* (Vintage Books, 1983).

Chapter Four

1. Centers for Disease Control, "Preliminary Report: Food-borne Outbreak of *Escherichia coli*," *Morbidity and Mortality Weekly Report*, Atlanta, February 5, 1993, pp. 85–86. (Hereafter CDC, *MMWR*.)

2. I deliberately leave aside until chapter 6 those powers of market access regulation that bear directly on public health. For a useful discussion, see Larry Gostin, "Traditional Public Health Strategies," in Harlon L. Dalton, Scott Burris, and the Yale AIDS Project, *AIDS and the Law: A Guide for the Public* (Yale University Press, 1987), pp. 47–65.

3. David F. Musto, "Quarantine and the Problem of AIDS," in Elizabeth Fee and Daniel M. Fox, eds., *AIDS: The Burdens of History* (University of California Press, 1988), p. 67. As Musto noted, the term comes from the Italian word

for "forty days" (*quarantina*), which "refers to the period during which ships capable of carrying contagious disease, such as plague, were kept isolated on their arrival at a seaport." Strictly speaking, a distinction exists between isolation and quarantine. The former separates infected persons from others during a period of communicability to prevent transmission of an infectious agent. The latter means detaining apparently healthy individuals for a period sufficient to ensure the absence of infection. See Gostin, "Traditional Public Health," p. 59.

4. See Musto, "Quarantine," p. 69.

5. Mark Caldwell, *The Last Crusade: The War on Consumption*, 1862-1954 (Atheneum, 1988).

6. Frank Ryan, *The Forgotten Plague: How the Battle against Tuberculosis Was Won—And Lost* (Little, Brown and Company, 1993).

7. Frank P. Grad, *Public Health Law Manual*, 2d ed. (Washington: American Public Health Association, 1990), p. 74.

8. 21 C.F.R. 1240.40.

9. 21 C.F.R. 1240.50.

10. CDC, "Summary of Notifiable Diseases, United States—1990," *MMWR*, October 4, 1991, p. 55.

11. 42 C.F.R. 71.32.

12. Joshua Lederberg, Robert E. Shope, and Stanley C. Oaks, Jr., eds., *Emerging Infections: Microbial Threats to Health in the United States* (Washington: National Academy Press, 1992), pp. 21—23.

13. Ibid., p. 23.

14. Ibid.

15. Telephone interview with Tony D. Perez, chief, Program Operations Branch, Division of Quarantine, CDC, Atlanta, June 21, 1993.

16. William Booth, "Cholera's Mysterious Journey North," *Washington Post*, August 26, 1991, p. A3.

17. Lederberg, Shope, and Oaks, *Emerging Infections*, p. 107.

18. CDC, "Pneumonic Plague—Arizona, 1992," *MMWR*, October 9, 1992, p. 738. See also Macfarlane Burnet and David O. White, *Natural History of Infectious Disease*, 4th ed. (Cambridge University Press, 1972), pp. 230—31.

19. A chilling overview of the potential hazard posed by these viruses is Richard Preston, "Crisis in the Hot Zone," *New Yorker*, October 26, 1992, pp. 58—80.

20. I have borrowed the term "alliance of terror" from Ryan, *The Forgotten Plague*, chap. 22.

21. The material in the paragraph draws from CDC, "National Action Plan to Combat Multidrug-Resistant Tuberculosis," *MMWR*, June 19, 1992, pp. 5—8, 54.

22. See ibid., p. 7, and later remarks by CDC officer Margarita E. Villarino, "Epidemiology of Recent TB Outbreaks and Implications for Drug Therapy," presentation to meeting of the American Public Health Association, Washington, D.C., November 9, 1992.

23. Ryan, *The Forgotten Plague*, p. 401.

24. CDC, "Tuberculosis Control Laws in the United States: A Survey and Recommendations," draft document, Atlanta, September 30, 1992.

25. Mireya Navarro, "New York City to Detain Patients Who Fail to Finish TB Treatment," *New York Times*, March 10, 1993, pp. A1, B4.

26. Cited in Albert R. Jonsen and Jeff Stryker, eds., *The Social Impact of AIDS in the United States* (Washington: National Academy Press, 1993), p. 36.

27. Ibid. A more detailed and up-to-date presentation of this research is Ronald Bayer and Amy Fairchild-Carrino, "AIDS and the Limits of Control: Public Health Orders, Quarantines, and Recalcitrant Behavior," *American Journal of Public Health*, vol. 83 (October 1993), pp. 1471–76.

28. Thomas R. Frieden and others, "The Emergence of Drug-Resistant Tuberculosis in New York City," *New England Journal of Medicine*, February 25, 1993, pp. 521–26; and Marian Goble and others, "Treatment of 171 Patients with Pulmonary Tuberculosis Resistant to Isoniazid and Rifampin," *New England Journal of Medicine*, February 25, 1993, pp. 527–32.

29. Goble and others, "Treatment of 171 Patients," p. 530.

30. Note that a major Supreme Court decision, *School Board of Nassau County v. Arline*, 480 U.S. 273 (1987), explicitly recognizes communicable disease (in this case, the tuberculosis suffered by a Florida teacher) as an impairment that might trigger prohibited discrimination. See Arthur S. Leonard, "Discrimination," in Scott Burris, Harlon L. Dalton, Judith Leonie Miller, and the Yale AIDS Project, eds., *AIDS Law Today: A New Guide for the Public* (Yale University Press, 1993), pp. 299–300.

31. This episode and the political history of the immigration ban are discussed in Robert M. Wachter, *The Fragile Coalition: Scientists, Activists and AIDS* (St. Martin's Press, 1991), chap. 4.

32. "Immigrants Infected with AIDS," *New York Times*, February 20, 1993, sec. 1, p. 18.

33. 56 Fed. Reg. 2484-86 (1991).

34. Letter to the editor from Lawrence O. Gostin, *New York Times*, March 4, 1993, p. A24.

35. Ibid.; and letter to the editor from John S. James, *New York Times*, March 4, 1993, p. A24.

36. For an extended criticism of both federal agency reliance on mandatory testing and the rationale for an immigration ban, see Donna I. Dennis, "HIV Screening and Discrimination: The Federal Example," in Burris and others, *AIDS Law Today: A New Guide for the Public*, pp. 187–215.

37. State and local health departments routinely screen refugees for tuberculosis, hepatitis B, and other pathogens. The federal government has subsidized this activity since 1985. See CDC, "Screening for Hepatitis B Virus Infection among Refugees Arriving in the United States, 1979–1991," *MMWR*, November 15, 1991, pp. 784–85.

38. Cristine Russell, "Ticked Off at Lyme Disease," *Washington Post*, July 14, 1992, p. Z12.

39. Robert A. Aronowitz, "Lyme Disease: The Social Construction of a New Disease and Its Social Consequences," *Milbank Quarterly,* vol. 69, no. 1 (1991), pp. 79–112.

40. Jonsen and Stryker, *The Social Impact of AIDS,* chap. 1.

41. Ronald Bayer, *Private Acts, Social Consequences: AIDS and the Politics of Public Health* (Free Press, 1989).

42. See Jonsen and Stryker, *The Social Impact of AIDS,* chap. 2. See also Stephen C. Joseph, *Dragon within the Gates: The Once and Future AIDS Epidemic* (Carroll and Graf, 1992); and Franklyn N. Judson and Thomas M. Vernon, Jr., "The Impact of AIDS on State and Local Health Departments: Issues and a Few Answers," *American Journal of Public Health,* vol. 78 (April 1988), pp. 387–93.

43. The immunoelectro transfer blot (Western Blot) also became the accepted method for confirming positive ELISA results.

44. Jonsen and Stryker, *The Social Impact of AIDS,* p. 27.

45. This paragraph relies on Bayer, *Private Acts, Social Consequences,* pp. 118–22.

46. Bayer, *Private Acts, Social Consequences,* pp. 121–22.

47. CDC, "Additional Recommendations to Reduce Sexual and Drug Abuse-Related Transmission of Human T-Lymphotropic Virus Type III," *MMWR,* March 14, 1986, p. 155.

48. Joseph, *Dragon,* p. 102.

49. Judson and Vernon, "The Impact of AIDS," pp. 388–89.

50. Ibid., pp. 389–90; Bayer, *Private Acts, Social Consequences,* chap. 2; and Joseph, *Dragon,* pp. 59–62.

51. Charles Backstrom and Leonard Robins, *The Minnesota Response to AIDS* (University of Minnesota, Center for Urban and Regional Affairs, 1992), pp. 2, 10–12.

52. Bruce Lambert, "U.S. Is Urging Vast Effort to Treat Million People Infected with AIDS Virus," *New York Times,* July 9, 1989, p. 25.

53. This paragraph draws on Bayer, *Private Acts, Social Consequences,* pp. 126–34.

54. Special Initiative on AIDS, *Contact Tracing and Partner Notification,* APHA/SIA Rept. 2 (Washington: American Public Health Association, November 1988), p. 5.

55. Bayer, *Private Acts, Social Consequences,* pp. 129–31. See also Kathleen E. Toomey and Willard Cates, Jr., "Partner Notification for the Prevention of HIV Infection," *AIDS,* vol. 3 (suppl. 1) (1989), p. S57.

56. Special Initiative on AIDS, *Contact Tracing,* p. 6.

57. Ibid., p. 6.

58. Ibid., p. 7.

59. Toomey and Cates, "Partner Notification," p. S58.

60. 53 Fed. Reg. 3554-58 (1988).

61. CDC, Division of STD/HIV Prevention, *Annual Report—1992,* p. 81.

62. CDC, Division of STD/HIV Prevention, *Annual Report*—1989, pp. 108, 110.

63. On the development of the military's HIV screening policy, see Bayer, *Private Acts, Social Consequences*, pp. 158—60; and Rhonda R. Rivera, "The Military," in Dalton, Burris, and Yale, *AIDS Law Project*, pp. 221—34.

64. General Accounting Office, *Defense Health Care: Effects of AIDS in the Military*, GAO/HRD-90-39 (Washington, February 1990), p. 13.

65. Bayer, *Private Acts, Social Consequences*, pp. 160—62.

66. Ibid., p. 159.

67. Ibid., pp. 158—62.

68. "When to Test for AIDS," editorial, *New York Times*, May 17, 1987, sec. 4, p. 26; and "More Testing Is Needed against AIDS Threat," letter to the editor from William J. Bennett, *New York Times*, June 1, 1987, p. A16.

69. Philip M. Boffey, "Reagan Urges Wide AIDS Testing but Does Not Call for Compulson," *New York Times*, June 1, 1987, pp. A1, A15.

70. Bayer, *Private Acts, Social Consequences*, p. 166.

71. National Organizations Responding to AIDS, "Mandatory Testing of Prisoners: The *AIDS Federal Policy Act*, H.R. 5142—Briefing Book," AIDS Action Council, Washington, D.C., 1988.

72. Isabel Wilkerson, "Prenuptial Tests for AIDS Repealed," *New York Times*, June 24, 1989, p. 6.

73. George A. Gellert and others, "Disclosure of AIDS," *New England Journal of Medicine*, November 5, 1992, p. 1389.

74. Calvin Sims, "H.I.V. Tests Up 60% since the Disclosure from Magic Johnson," *New York Times*, December 7, 1991, pp. 1, 28.

75. David L. Cohn and others, "Denver's Increase in HIV Counseling after Magic Johnson's HIV Disclosure," letter, *American Journal of Public Health*, vol. 82 (December 1992), p. 1692.

76. See Gellert and others, "Disclosure of AIDS." See also Amy Fairchild Carrino and Ronald Bayer, "More on Disclosure of AIDS in Celebrities," *New England Journal of Medicine*, February 25, 1993, p. 583.

77. Jay Mathews, "Surge in AIDS Tests Drying Up Budgets," *Washington Post*, December 22, 1991, p. A3. In a similar though more restricted development, the revelation that world featherweight boxing champion Ruben Palacio had tested positive for HIV and been stripped of his title set off a surge of testing in the boxing community. "Fanfare: AIDS Testing on Upswing," *Washington Post*, April 22, 1993, p. B2.

78. CDC, "Possible Transmission of Human Immunodeficiency Virus to a Patient during an Invasive Dental Procedure," *MMWR*, July 27, 1990, pp. 489—93.

79. "Hospital Offers Tests after Surgeon Dies of AIDS," *New York Times*, December 3, 1990, p. A20; and Susan Okie, "Johns Hopkins Hospital Seeks New AIDS Guidelines," *Washington Post*, December 15, 1990, p. A5.

80. CDC, "Update: Transmission of HIV Infection during an Invasive Dental Procedure—Florida," *MMWR*, January 18, 1991, pp. 21—27, 33. Quotation on p. 27.

81. For a thorough analysis of this issue with regard to federalism, see Mark Rom, "Health-Care Workers and HIV: Policy Choice in a Federal System," *Publius*, vol. 23 (Summer 1993), pp. 135–53.

82. Malcolm Gladwell, "HIV-Infected Doctors Fear They Are Targets," *Washington Post*, April 2, 1991, p. A1. The polling results are in Barbara Kantrowitz and others, "Doctors and AIDS," *Newsweek*, July 1, 1991, p. 52.

83. Lawrence K. Altman, "U.S. Hears Debate on Mandatory AIDS Tests for Health Workers," *New York Times*, February 22, 1991, p. A15.

84. Malcolm Gladwell, "Groups Oppose HIV Tests for Medical Professionals," *Washington Post*, February 22, 1991, p. A6.

85. Nicholas Hentoff, "Doctors with AIDS," *Washington Post*, December 28, 1990, p. A19; and "Public Health Doesn't Gain from AIDS Education: For Mandatory Testing," letter to the editor from Sanford F. Kuvin, *New York Times*, January 23, 1991, p. A18.

86. Lawrence K. Altman, "AIDS-Infected Doctors and Dentists Are Urged to Warn Patients or Quit," *New York Times*, January 18, 1991, p. A18.

87. Philip J. Hilts, "AIDS Patient Urges Congress to Pass Testing Bill," *New York Times*, September 27, 1991, p. A12.

88. Martin Tolchin, "Senate Adopts Tough Measures on Health Workers with AIDS," *New York Times*, July 19, 1991, pp. A1, A14.

89. *Congressional Record*, daily ed., July 18, 1991, p. S10333.

90. Malcolm Gladwell, "HIV Tests in the Health Profession," *Washington Post*, September 11, 1991, p. A21.

91. Tolchin, "Senate Adopts Tough Measures," p. A1.

92. CDC, "Recommendations for Preventing Transmission of Human Immunodeficiency Virus and Hepatitis B Virus to Patients during Exposure-Prone Invasive Procedures," *MMWR*, July 12, 1991.

93. Ibid., p. 6.

94. Ibid., pp. 5–6.

95. *Congressional Record*, daily ed., October 2, 1991, p. H7311. This legislative language was drafted to make such a funding termination exceedingly unlikely, as the HHS secretary could "extend the time period for a State, upon application of such State, that additional time is required for instituting said guidelines."

96. Jane S. Smith, *Patenting the Sun: Polio and the Salk Vaccine* (William Morrow, 1990); and Donald R. Hopkins, *Princes and Peasants: Smallpox in History* (University of Chicago Press, 1983).

97. Harry F. Dowling, *Fighting Infection: Conquests of the Twentieth Century* (Harvard University Press, 1977).

98. One familiar informational vehicle is the federal Advisory Committee on Immunization Practices, whose recommendations are regularly and widely disseminated among health providers.

99. A comprehensive overview of these activities is contained in the annual justification material submitted to the congressional appropriations committees. See *Departments of Labor, Health and Human Services, Education and Related Agencies Appropriations for 1993*, Hearings before the Subcommittee on the Departments of Labor, Health and Human Services, Education and Related

Agencies of the House Committee on Appropriations, 102 Cong. 2 sess. (GPO, 1992), pp. 1641–1779.

100. Ibid., p. 1451.

101. Ibid., pp. 1438–44, 1717.

102. Interview with Barbara Levine, American Public Health Association, Washington, D.C., October 5, 1992.

103. Richard E. Neustadt and Harvey V. Fineberg, *The Epidemic That Never Was: Policy-Making and the Swine Flu Scare* (Vintage Books, 1983); Arthur M. Silverstein, *Pure Politics and Impure Science: The Swine Flu Affair* (Johns Hopkins University Press, 1981); Diana B. Dutton, "The Swine Flu Immunization Program," in *Worse than the Disease: Pitfalls of Medical Progress* (Cambridge University Press, 1988), chap. 5; and Joseph A. Califano, Jr., *Governing America: An Insider's Report from the White House and the Cabinet* (Simon and Schuster, 1981), pp. 172–78.

104. Peter S. Arno and Karyn L. Feiden, *Against the Odds: The Story of AIDS Drug Development, Politics, and Profits* (Harper Collins, 1992), chap. 11.

Chapter Five

1. Frank P. Grad, *The Public Health Law Manual*, 2d ed. (Washington: American Public Health Association, 1990), p. 73.

2. Data for the 1980s demonstrate a sharp decline in DTP only in 1984 in the wake of vaccine shortage. See Walter A. Orenstein and Roger H. Bernier, "Surveillance in the Control of Vaccine-Preventable Diseases," in William Halperin, Edward L. Baker, Jr., and Richard R. Monson, eds., *Public Health Surveillance* (Van Nostrand Reinhold, 1992), p. 88.

3. For an excellent overview, see Charles F. Turner, Heather G. Miller, and Lincoln E. Moses, eds., *AIDS: Sexual Behavior and Intravenous Drug Use* (Washington: National Academy Press, 1989).

4. Marshall H. Becker and Jill G. Joseph, "AIDS and Behavioral Change to Reduce Risk: A Review," *American Journal of Public Health*, vol. 78 (April 1988), pp. 394–410.

5. Becker and Joseph, "AIDS," p. 407.

6. Ibid., p. 403; and Turner, Miller, and Moses, *AIDS: Sexual Behavior and Intravenous Drug Use*, p. 261. See also Don C. Des Jarlais and Samuel R. Friedman, "AIDS and the Use of Injected Drugs," *Scientific American*, vol. 270 (February 1994), pp. 82–88.

7. R. E. Chaisson and others, "Human Immunodeficiency Virus Infection in Heterosexual Intravenous Drug Users in San Francisco," *American Journal of Public Health*, vol. 77 (February 1987), pp. 169–72.

8. Sandra G. Boodman, "AIDS Risk Looms over Gays Ignoring Advice, Experts Say," *Washington Post*, November 22, 1987, pp. A1, A20, A21; and Bruce Lambert, "Relapses into Risky Sex Seen by AIDS Experts," *New York Times*, June 22, 1990, p. A18.

9. "Almost One-Third of Gay Men in Study Admit to Unprotected Anal Intercourse," *Washington Post*, November 19, 1992, p. A2. The problem was not

limited to the United States. For data on Amsterdam, see John B. F. de Wit and others, "Increase in Unprotected Anogenital Intercourse among Homosexual Men," *American Journal of Public Health*, vol. 83 (October 1993), pp. 1451–53.

10. David Gelman and others, "The Young and the Reckless," *Newsweek*, January 11, 1993, pp. 60–61.

11. Centers for Disease Control, "Condom Use and Sexual Identity among Men Who Have Sex with Men—Dallas, 1991," *Morbidity and Mortality Weekly Report*, Atlanta, January 15, 1993, pp. 7, 13. (Hereafter CDC, *MMWR*.)

12. Joseph A. Catania and others, "Prevalence of AIDS-Related Risk Factors and Condom Use in the United States," *Science*, November 13, 1992, pp. 1101–06; and Anke A. Ehrhardt, "Trends in Sexual Behavior and the HIV Pandemic," *American Journal of Public Health*, vol. 82 (November 1992), pp. 1459–61.

13. CDC, *MMWR*, January 29, 1993, p. 46. The survey does, however, identify a trend among "all race, sex and age groups" toward fewer "one-night stands."

14. Turner, Miller, and Moses, *AIDS: Sexual Behavior and Intravenous Drug Use*, pp. 262–63. See also Barbara Gerbert and Bryan Maguire, "Public Acceptance of the Surgeon General's Brochure on AIDS," *Public Health Reports*, vol. 104 (March–April 1989), pp. 130–33.

15. Turner, Miller, and Moses, *AIDS: Sexual Behavior and Intravenous Drug Use*, pp. 277–79; and Kenneth G. Castro, Ronald O. Valdiserri, and James W. Curran, "Perspectives on HIV/AIDS Epidemiology and Prevention from the Eighth International Conference on AIDS," *American Journal of Public Health*, vol. 82 (November 1992), p. 1467.

16. Turner, Miller, and Moses, *AIDS: Sexual Behavior and Intravenous Drug Use*, pp. 266–68.

17. Ibid., p. 286.

18. Ibid., pp. 283–85; and Becker and Joseph, "AIDS and Behavioral Change," p. 408.

19. Ronald Bayer, *Private Acts, Social Consequences: AIDS and the Politics of Public Health* (Free Press, 1989), chap. 7; and C. Everett Koop, *Koop: The Memoirs of America's Family Doctor* (Random House, 1991), chap. 9, provide helpful overviews.

20. Bayer, *Private Acts, Social Consequences*, p. 207.

21. Michael J. Fumento suggests that conservatives saw in the epidemic an opportunity to drive home their agenda of moral reconstruction. See "The Political Uses of an Epidemic," *New Republic*, August 8/15, 1988, pp. 19–23.

22. Bayer, *Private Acts, Social Consequences*, p. 212.

23. Robert D. McFadden, "Judge Overturns U.S. Rule Blocking 'Offensive' Educational Material on AIDS," *New York Times*, May 12, 1992, p. B3.

24. Quoted ibid.

25. Quotations are from letter by William McBeath to William L. Roper, CDC director, February 16, 1993.

26. Julie Kosterlitz, "AIDS Wars," *National Journal*, July 25, 1992, pp. 1727–32.

27. Malcolm Gladwell, "AIDS Education Effort Called Short on Facts," *Washington Post*, March 27, 1992, p. A19. See also Malcolm Gladwell, "A Matter

of Condom Sense," *Washington Post*, April 9, 1992, p. C1, C9; and Philip J. Hilts, "U.S. Agency Is Criticized for Dropping AIDS Ads," *New York Times*, July 1, 1992, p. A10.

28. Quoted in Turner, Miller, and Moses, *AIDS: Sexual Behavior and Intravenous Drug Use*, p. 377.

29. The final provision of Public Law 101-381 (104 Stat. 628), the Ryan White Comprehensive AIDS Resources Emergency Act of 1990, states that "none of the funds made available under this Act, or an amendment made by this Act, shall be used to provide individuals with hypodermic needles or syringes so that such individuals may use illegal drugs." See 104 Stat. 628. On the politics of needle exchange in New York and elsewhere, see Stephen C. Joseph, *Dragon within the Gates: The Once and Future AIDS Epidemic* (Carroll and Graf, 1992), chap. 8; and Bayer, *Private Acts, Social Consequences*, pp. 218–25.

30. Karen De Witt, "In U.S. Ads for TV, Condoms That Dare Speak Their Name," *New York Times*, January 5, 1994, pp. A1, A12; and Stuart Elliott, "Advertising: The Condom is the Star of the Government's New Anti-AIDS Spots," *New York Times*, p. D6.

31. CDC, "Recommendations for Preventing Transmissions of Human Immunodeficiency Virus and Hepatitis B Virus to Patients during Exposure-Prone Invasive Procedures," *MMWR*, July 12, 1991, p. 5.

32. Malcolm Gladwell, "Medical Groups Reject Limits on HIV-Infected Workers," *Washington Post*, November 5, 1991, pp. A1, A4.

33. "California Groups Rebuff AIDS-Risk List Request," *New York Times*, October 19, 1991, sec. 1, p. 7.

34. Gladwell, "Medical Groups Reject Limits on HIV-Infected Workers," p. A4; and "C.D.C. to List Operations as AIDS Risks," *New York Times*, November 6, 1991, p. C17.

35. Lawrence K. Altman, "U.S. Backs Off on Plan to Restrict Health Workers with AIDS Virus," *New York Times*, December 4, 1991, pp. A1, C19; and Warren E. Leary, "A.M.A. Backs Off on an AIDS Risk List," *New York Times*, December 15, 1991, sec. 1, p. 38.

36. Altman, "U.S. Backs Off."

37. Karen M. Starko and others, "Reye's Syndrome and Salicylate Use," *Pediatrics*, vol. 66 (December 1980), pp. 859–64.

38. CDC, "National Surveillance for Reye Syndrome, 1981," *MMWR*, February 12, 1982, p. 54.

39. Ibid., p. 55.

40. Elizabeth W. Etheridge, *Sentinel for Health: A History of the Centers for Disease Control* (University of California Press, 1992), pp. 297–98.

41. CDC, *MMWR*, February 12, 1982, p. 55.

42. American Academy of Pediatrics, draft "news and comment" release, EIR Grove Village, Illinois, December 1, 1981.

43. Letter from Sidney M. Wolfe, director, Public Citizen Health Research Group, to Mark Novitch, associate commissioner, Food and Drug Administration (FDA), March 9, 1982.

44. CDC, "Surgeon General's Advisory on the Use of Salicylates and Reye Syndrome," *MMWR*, June 11, 1982, p. 289.

45. Michael de Courcy Hinds, "Warning Issued on Giving Aspirin to Children," *New York Times*, June 5, 1982, p. A1.

46. "U.S. Seeks New Study on Reye's Syndrome," *New York Times*, November 19, 1982, p. A18.

47. Tim Miller, "The O.M.B. Writes a Prescription," *The Nation*, March 31, 1984, p. 383.

48. In July 1984 the United States Court of Appeals for the D.C. Circuit concluded that the record "strongly suggests that the pace of agency decision-making is unreasonably dilatory," that "all scientific evidence in the record points to a link between [aspirin] and Reye's Syndrome," and that industry's role in the delay was troubling given that "the pace of agency decision-making may jeopardize the lives of children." Quoted in Public Citizen, *Risking America's Health and Safety: George Bush and the Task Force on Regulatory Relief* (Washington, 1988), p. 9.

49. Boyce Rensberger, "FDA Attacks Pro-Aspirin Ad," *Washington Post*, November 6, 1984, p. A1.

50. FDA press release, January 25, 1985, in *FDA Issues*, Hearings before the Subcommittee on Health and the Environment of the House Committee on Energy and Commerce, 99 Cong. 1 sess. (GPO, 1985), p. 381.

51. Public Citizen also sought to have the Federal Trade Commission invoke its authority to prohibit "unfair and deceptive" business practices to require a strong warning label. See letter from Sidney Wolfe and Katherine A. Meyer to James C. Miller III, chairman, Federal Trade Commission, January 16, 1985.

52. *FDA Issues*, Hearings, p. 276. While Schering-Plough had negotiated separately, their labeling proposal could be perceived as possibly more explicit and aggressive than that to which the foundation members agreed. See pp. 381–82.

53. Ibid., pp. 276–77.

54. Ibid., p. 279.

55. See, for example, Philip M. Boffey, "Study Reported to Tighten Link of Aspirin and Reye's Syndrome," *New York Times*, January 9, 1985, p. A14.

56. Cited in "FDA Orders Warning of Reye's Syndrome for Aspirin Bottles," *Washington Post*, March 8, 1986, p. A8.

57. "Delay on Aspirin Warning Label Cost Children's Lives, Study Says," *New York Times*, October 23, 1992, p. A12.

58. CDC, *MMWR*, May 23, 1980, pp. 229–30, and June 27, 1980, pp. 297–99.

59. *Toxic Shock Syndrome, 1980*, Hearing before the Subcommittee on Health and Scientific Research of the Senate Committee on Labor and Human Resources, 96 Cong. 2 sess. (GPO, 1980); and Marcia E. Donawa, George R. Schmid, and Michael T. Osterholm, "Toxic Shock Syndrome: Chronology of State and Federal Epidemiologic Studies and Regulatory Decision-Making," *Public Health Reports*, vol. 99 (July–August 1984), pp. 342–50.

60. See 45 Fed. Reg. 12715-18 (1980). No performance standard for any class II device would emerge until much later. See Christopher H. Foreman, Jr.,

Signals from the Hill: Congressional Oversight and the Challenge of Social Regulation (Yale University Press, 1988), pp. 51–53.

61. Letter to Dr. Patrick G. Laing from F. Alan Andersen, acting associate director for standards, Bureau of Medical Devices, FDA, July 13, 1981.

62. Letter to F. Alan Andersen, Bureau of Medical Devices, FDA, from Wayne Ellis, chairman pro-tempore, Committee F-4 Task Force on Tampons, January 22, 1982.

63. M. T. Osterholm and others, "Tri-State Toxic-Shock Syndrome Study. I. Epidemiologic Findings," *Journal of Infectious Diseases*, vol. 145 (April 1982) pp. 431–40.

64. 47 Fed. Reg. 26982 (1982).

65. Letter to Arthur Hull Hayes, FDA Commissioner, from Allen Greenberg and Sidney M. Wolfe, Public Citizen, Washington, D.C., July 29, 1982.

66. Letter to Sidney M. Wolfe and Allen Greenberg, Public Citizen, from Mark Novitch, acting commissioner of food and drugs, September 22, 1982.

67. Letter to Mark Novitch, acting commissioner, FDA, from Allen Greenberg and Sidney Wolfe, May 7, 1984.

68. Interview with Patti Goldman, Public Citizen Litigation Group, Washington, D.C., December 21, 1989.

69. Letter to Allen Greenberg, Health Research Group, from John C. Villforth, director, Center for Devices and Radiological Health, FDA, July 9, 1984.

70. See "Memorandum in Support of Plaintiffs' Motion for Summary Judgment," Public Citizen, Washington, 1988, p. 7, and exhibit 11 of plaintiff's exhibits.

71. Letter to Frank E. Young, FDA commissioner, from Sidney M. Wolfe and Pauline Sobel, Public Citizen Health Research Group, Washington, D.C., August 20, 1987. The epidemiologic study is Seth F. Berkeley and others, "The Relationship of Tampon Characteristics to Menstrual Toxic Shock Syndrome," *Journal of the American Medical Association*, August 21, 1987, pp. 917–20.

72. 53 Fed. Reg. 37250-67 (1988).

73. See Comments of Playtex Family Products to FDA's proposed rule for tampon absorbency labeling, December 20, 1988, pp. 3–4, 23. (Docket No. 86-N-0479), Dockets Management Branch, FDA, Rockville, Md.

74. *Public Citizen Health Research Group et al. v. Commissioner, Food and Drug Administration et al.*, 724 F. Supp. 1013 (D.C. 1989).

75. 54 Fed. Reg. 43766-75 (1989).

76. CDC, "Summary of Notifiable Diseases, United States, 1991," *MMWR*, October 2, 1992, p. 57.

77. Remarks by Dr. Paula Fujiwara, CDC official attached to the New York City Bureau of TB Control, before the American Public Health Association, Washington, D.C., November 9, 1992, and telephone interview, November 24, 1992.

78. See Anthony Downs, *Inside Bureaucracy* (Little, Brown, 1967), p. 33, and Alan Stone *Regulation and Its Alternatives* (CQ Press, 1982), p. 85.

79. Susan L. Coyle, Robert F. Boruch, and Charles F. Turner, eds., *Evaluating AIDS Prevention Programs* (Washington: National Academy Press, 1991).

80. David G. Ostrow, "AIDS Prevention through Effective Education," *Daedalus*, vol. 118 (Summer 1989), pp. 240–41.

81. Office of Technology Assessment, *How Effective Is AIDS Education?* (GPO, May 1988).

Chapter Six

1. Although information control is often considered regulation, it is an *educational* mechanism in this volume.

2. *Food, Drug, Cosmetic, and Device Enforcement Amendments*, Hearing before the Subcommittee on Health and the Environment of the House Committee on Energy and Commerce, 102 Cong. 1 sess. (Government Printing Office, 1991); and John Carey, "The FDA May Soon Be Able to Back Up Its Snarl," *Business Week*, October 28, 1991, p. 40.

3. This information is contained in General Accounting Office, *FDA's Oversight of the 1982 Canned Salmon Recalls*, GAO/HRD-84-77 (Washington, September 1984); and quoted in Comptroller General, *Legislative Changes and Administrative Improvements Should Be Considered for FDA to Better Protect the Public from Adulterated Food Products*, GAO/HRD-84-61 (Washington, September 1984), p. 39. Emphasis added.

4. Comptroller General, *Legislative Changes*, p. 10.

5. GAO, *FDA's Oversight*, p. 1.

6. Ibid.

7. *Deficiencies in FDA's Regulation of the Marketing of Unapproved New Drugs: The Case of E-Ferol*, H. Rept. 98-1168, 98 Cong. 2 sess. (GPO, 1984).

8. Ibid., p. 6.

9. For example, between fiscal years 1983 and 1988, the Food and Drug Administration (FDA) oversaw recalls of 1,635 different medical devices, with 48 of the recalls serious enough to warrant a Class I designation. See GAO, *Medical Device Recalls: An Overview and Analysis 1983–88*, GAO/PEMD-89-15BR (Washington, August 1989), p. 1.

10. On the politics of the polio vaccine, see Jane S. Smith, *Patenting the Sun: Polio and the Salk Vaccine* (Doubleday, 1990), esp. pp. 366–68, on the Cutter incident.

11. "Bon Vivant's Canned Food Is Being Recalled by U.S.," *New York Times*, July, 8, 1971, p. 1.

12. "Bon Vivant Files for Bankruptcy," *New York Times*, July 27, 1971, p. 40. This episode is unusual in that the offending firm's entire product line quickly became suspect and subject to withdrawal, hence the bankruptcy.

13. Richard D. Lyons, "Budget Doubling Sought by F.D.A.," *New York Times*, September 11, 1971, p. 18.

14. Timothy Egan, "Tainted Hamburger Raises Doubts on Meat Safety," *New York Times*, January 27, 1993, p. A10; and Carole Sugarman, "Espy to Seek New U.S. Meat Inspection System," *Washington Post*, February 6, 1993, p. A5.

15. On this point, see Paul J. Quirk, "Food and Drug Administration," in James Q. Wilson, ed., *The Politics of Regulation* (Basic Books, 1980), pp. 192–201.

16. On the importance of the scope of conflict, see E. E. Schattschneider, *The Semisovereign People* (Holt, Rinehart and Winston, 1960).

17. Stephen Koepp, "A Hard Decision to Swallow," *Time*, March 3, 1986, p. 59.

18. See the testimony of Joseph P. Hile, FDA associate commissioner for regulatory affairs, *Health and the Environment—Part 1*, Hearings before the Subcommittee on Health and the Environment of the House Committee on Energy and Commerce, 98 Cong. 1 sess. (GPO, 1983), p. 19.

19. *Tamper-Resistant Packaging for Over-the-Counter Drugs*, Hearing before the Subcommittee on Health and the Environment of the House Committee on Energy and Commerce, 97 Cong. 2 sess. (GPO, 1982), p. 7.

20. Ibid., p. 23.

21. Ibid., p. 22.

22. Harold Hopkins, "Relief in Tamper-Resistant Packages," *FDA Consumer*, vol. 17 (February 1983), p. 13.

23. *The Federal Anti-Tampering Act*, S. Rept. 98-69, 98 Cong. 1 sess. (GPO, 1983), p. 6.

24. Ibid., p. 5.

25. Cristine Russell, "Putting a Lid on Product Tampering," *Washington Post*, May 23, 1986, p. A13; and Malcolm Gladwell, "Poisoning Cases Prompt Recall of 12-Hour Sudafed Capsules," *Washington Post*, March 4, 1991, pp. A1, A5.

26. Bill Powell, "The Tylenol Rescue," *Newsweek*, March 8, 1986, pp. 52–53.

27. *Human Resources Impact: Over-the Counter Product Packaging Safety*, Hearing before the Senate Committee on Labor and Human Resources, 99 Cong. 2 sess. (GPO, 1986).

28. This account draws heavily on Gerald Astor, *The Disease Detectives: Deadly Medical Mysteries and the People Who Solved Them* (New American Library, 1983), pp. 200–02; and *Infant Formula: Our Children Need Better Protection*, Committee Print 96-IFC 42, 96 Cong. 2 sess. (GPO, 1980). See also Christopher J. Foreman, Jr., *Signals from the Hill: Congressional Oversight and the Challenge of Social Regulation* (Yale University Press, 1988), pp. 47–48.

29. *Infant Formula*, Hearing before the Subcommittee on Oversight and Investigations of the House Committee on Interstate and Foreign Commerce, 96 Cong. 1 sess. (GPO, 1980).

30. *Infant Formula: The Present Danger*, Hearing before the Subcommittee on Oversight and Investigations of the House Committee on Energy and Commerce, 97 Cong. 2 sess. (GPO, 1982).

31. On the quality control regulation, see 47 Fed. Reg. 17016-27 (1982). On the recall requirements, see 47 Fed. Reg. 18832-36 (1982).

32. Lester B. Lave, *The Strategy of Social Regulation: Decision Frameworks for Policy* (Brookings, 1981), pp. 17–19.

33. Ibid., pp. 11–13.

34. Richard E. Neustadt and Harvey V. Fineberg, *The Epidemic That Never Was: Policy-Making and the Swine Flu Scare* (Vintage Books, 1983), p. 95.

35. The material in these paragraphs is taken from Ibid., pp. 91–97.

36. *Deficiencies in FDA's Regulation of the New Drug "Oraflex,"* H. Rept. 98-511, 98 Cong. 1 sess. (GPO, 1983); and *FDA's Regulation of Zomax,* H. Rept. 98-584, 98 Cong. 1 sess. (GPO, 1983).

37. Michael D. Lemonick, "Reprieve for Breast Implants," *Time,* November 25, 1991, p. 81; Jane Gross, "Women with Breast Implants Split on Need for U.S. Controls," *New York Times,* November 5, 1991, p. A1, A18; and Jane Gross, "What Now? Many Ask after Implant Decision," *New York Times,* January 8, 1992, p. A16.

38. Felicity Barringer, "First Steps Taken in Revived Use of Breast Implants," *New York Times,* May 3, 1992, p. 34.

39. Malcolm Gladwell, "FDA Will Allow Limited Use of Silicone-Gel Breast Implants," *Washington Post,* April 17, 1992, p. A2.

40. Laurence Slutsker and others, "Eosinophilia-Myalgia Syndrome Associated with Exposure to Tryptophan from a Single Manufacturer," *Journal of the American Medical Association,* July 11, 1990, pp. 213–17.

41. I rely heavily here on the reporting of Tamar Stieber, reprinted in Kendall J. Wills, ed., *The Pulitzer Prizes: 1990* (Simon and Schuster, 1990), pp. 451–80.

42. Ibid., p. 470.

43. The Code of Federal Regulations explains the concept in the following way: "It is impracticable to list all substances that are generally recognized as safe for their intended use. However, the [FDA] Commissioner regards such common food ingredients as salt, pepper, vinegar and baking powder, and monosodium glutamate as safe for their intended use" [so long as 'good manufacturing practice' prevails]. 21 C.F.R. Part 182, Subpart A, section 182.1(a).

44. 37 Fed. Reg. 6938 (1972).

45. For a full account of L-tryptophan's regulatory and political context, see *FDA's Regulation of the Dietary Supplement L-Tryptophan,* Hearing before the Subcommittee on Human Resources and Intergovernmental Relations of the House Committee on Government Operations, 102 Cong. 1 sess. (GPO, 1992). See also Malcolm Gladwell, "72 Diet-Pill Ban Ignored until Recent Deaths," *Washington Post,* September 5, 1990, pp. A1, A15.

46. See Public Law 94-278 (90 Stat. 410).

47. *Congressional Record,* daily ed., December 11, 1975, p. S39983.

48. See Gladwell, "'72 Diet-Pill Ban."

49. See especially the testimony of Richard J. Wurtman in *FDA's Regulation of the Dietary Supplement L-Tryptophan,* Hearing, pp. 70–76.

50. Malcolm Gladwell, "To Alan Morrison, Justice Falls Short in Robins Case," *Washington Post,* September 19, 1989, pp. C1, C2. The fullest chronicle of the episode is Morton Mintz, *At Any Cost: Corporate Greed, Women, and the Dalkon Shield* (Pantheon Books, 1985).

51. As early as 1968 an FDA advisory committee had found troubling signs of an inadequately regulated market for intrauterine devices. See Mintz, *At Any Cost,* p. 55.

52. Ibid., pp. 166–67.

53. "Dalkon Shield's Safety, Effectiveness Studied," *Public Health Reports,* vol. 90 (March–April 1975), p. 188.

54. Mintz, *At Any Cost*, p. 172.

55. Sanford L. Weiner, "Tampons and Toxic Shock Syndrome: Consumer Protection or Public Confusion?" in Harvey M. Sapolsky, ed., *Consuming Fears: The Politics of Product Risks* (Basic Books, 1986), pp. 149–53.

56. For a breakdown of the average times required for new drugs to make their way from the lab to the marketplace, see C. Vance Gordon and Dale E. Wierenga, "The Drug Development and Approval Process," in "New Drug Approvals in 1991," press release, Pharmaceutical Manufacturers Association, Washington, D.C., January 1992, p. 10.

57. See, for example, Peter Brimelow and Leslie Spencer, "Food and Drugs and Politics," *Forbes*, November 22, 1993, pp. 115–19.

58. See Sam Peltzman, *Regulation of Pharmaceutical Innovation: The 1962 Amendments* (Washington: American Enterprise Institute, 1974).

59. George C. Eads and Michael Fix, *Relief or Reform? Reagan's Regulatory Dilemma* (Washington: Urban Institute Press, 1984). Statutory revision was not one of the main avenues employed to pursue the Reagan regulatory agenda. Congressional opposition largely foreclosed that path, and congressional Democrats attacked the Reagan effort at every opportunity. See Christopher H. Foreman, Jr., "Legislators, Regulators, and the OMB: The Congressional Challenge to Presidential Regulatory Relief," in James A. Thurber, ed., *Divided Democracy: Cooperation and Conflict between the President and Congress* (Washington: Congressional Quarterly Press, 1991), pp. 123–43.

60. *AIDS Drugs: Where Are They?*, H. Rept. 100-1092, 100 Cong. 2 sess. (GPO, 1988). A careful reading of this report suggests that Chairman Weiss, while anxious to give AIDS activists a forum to ventilate their concerns and interested in seeing the broadest possible distribution of promising but unapproved drugs in the context of clinical trials, remained unwilling to embrace any radical overhaul of FDA practice. Instead, Weiss tended to blame the NIAID for failing to get enough drugs into the regulatory pipeline.

61. Gina Kolata, "Petition Seeks to Speed Approval of AIDS Drugs," *New York Times*, December 21, 1990, p. A31.

62. See David Ellen, "Testing, Testing," *New Republic*, August 28, 1989, pp. 14–15; and David Vogel, "AIDS and the Politics of Drug Lag," *Public Interest*, no. 96 (Summer 1989), pp. 73–85.

63. See statement before the National Commission on AIDS by Ellen C. Cooper, director, division of antiviral drug products, FDA, May 7, 1990. The lack of a level playing field among AIDS drug developers is criticized in Bruce Nussbaum, *Good Intentions: How Big Business and the Medical Establishment Are Corrupting the Fight Against AIDS* (Atlantic Monthly Press, 1990).

64. *AIDS Treatment Research and Approval*, Hearing before the Senate Committee on Labor and Human Resources, 100 Cong. 2 sess. (GPO, 1988), p. 72.

65. 53 Fed. Reg. 41516 (1988).

66. Ibid., p. 41523.

67. *AIDS Drugs: Where Are They?*, H. Rept. 100-1092, p. 28.

68. 55 Fed. Reg. 20857 (1990).

69. National Association of People with AIDS, *Medical Alert*, vol. 1 (January 1993), p. 1. See also interview with David Feigal, director, division of antiviral drug products, FDA, in *AIDS Treatment News*, May 21, 1993.

70. John Schwartz, "FDA Clears 4th Drug to Fight AIDS," *Washington Post*, June 28, 1994, p. A12.

71. Gina Kolata, "Private Doctors Testing New Drugs in Novel Approach," *New York Times*, July 9, 1989, p. A1.

72. Jeffrey Levi, "The Availability of Unproven AIDS Therapies: FDA and DDI," paper prepared for Institute of Medicine, Washington, D.C., 1990.

73. Gina Kolata, "Interest Grows in Licensing Shortcut for 2 AIDS Drugs," *New York Times*, September 25, 1990, p. C3.

74. *AIDS Drugs: Where Are They?*, H. Rept. 100-1092, p. 29.

75. See, for example, George J. Annas, "Faith (Healing), Hope, and Charity at the FDA: The Politics of AIDS Drug Trials," in Lawrence O. Gostin, ed., *AIDS and the Health Care System* (Yale University Press, 1990), pp. 183–94.

76. Mireya Navarro, "Hemophiliacs Demand Answers as AIDS Toll Rises," *New York Times*, May 10, 1993, pp. A1, B2; and Eliot Marshall, "The Politics of Breast Cancer," *Science*, January 29, 1993, pp. 616–17.

77. William F. West, *Administrative Rulemaking: Politics and Processes* (Greenwood Press, 1985).

78. This is more likely in traditional price-and-entry regulation than in the health and safety area, where public alarm through media attention is easier to create.

79. *Reports on AIDS Published in the Morbidity and Mortality Weekly Report—June 1981 through May 1986* (Atlanta: Centers for Disease Control, 1986), p. 14. (Hereafter *Reports on AIDS*.)

80. Ibid., pp. 24–26.

81. Ibid., pp. 26–27.

82. *Report of the Presidential Commission on the Human Immunodeficiency Virus Epidemic* (Washington, June 1988), p. 78.

83. Ibid. Other critical assessments of this response include: Charles Perrow and Mauro F. Guillén, *The AIDS Disaster: The Failure of Organizations in New York and the Nation* (Yale University Press, 1990), pp. 38–44; Gilbert M. Gaul, "The Loose Way the FDA Regulates Blood Industry," in Kendall J. Wills, ed., *The Pulitzer Prizes: 1990* (Simon and Schuster, 1990), pp. 53–67; Ross D. Eckert, "AIDS and the Blood Bankers," *Regulation*, vol. 10 (September–October 1986), pp. 15–24; Ross D. Eckert and Edward L. Wallace, *Securing a Safer Blood Supply: Two Views* (Washington: American Enterprise Institute, 1985), chap. 5; and Harvey M. Sapolsky and Stephen L. Boswell, "The History of Transfusion AIDS: Practice and Policy Alternatives," in Elizabeth Fee and Daniel M. Fox, eds., *AIDS: The Making of a Chronic Disease* (University of California Press, 1992), pp. 170–93.

84. *Blood Supply Safety*, Hearing before the Subcommittee on Oversight and Investigations of the House Committee on Energy and Commerce, 101 Cong. 2 sess. (GPO, 1990), p. 45.

85. Randy Shilts, *And the Band Played On: Politics, People, and the AIDS Epidemic* (St. Martin's Press, 1987), pp. 207, 220, 224, 242.

86. Quoted in Eckert and Wallace, *Securing*, p. 61. See also Perrow and Guillén, *The AIDS Disaster*, p. 39.

87. Quoted in the statement of Ross D. Eckert in *Blood Supply Safety*, Hearing, p. 28. See also Shilts, *And the Band Played On*, p. 333.

88. Statement of Ross D. Eckert, *Blood Supply Safety*, Hearing, pp. 11–12.

89. *Blood Supply Safety*, Hearing, pp. 34–35.

90. 53 Fed. Reg. 111-17 (1988).

91. Gaul, "The Loose Way," p. 54.

92. Office of Technology Assessment, *Blood Policy and Technology* (Washington, 1985), p. 5. See pp. 4–7 for a summary of the blood services industry's structure.

93. Eckert and Wallace, *Securing*, p. 61.

94. *Blood Supply Safety*, Hearing, pp. 29–30.

95. Robin Herman, "Continuing Vigilance over the Blood Supply," *Washington Post*, April 21, 1992, p. 28.

96. *Blood Supply Safety*, Hearing, p. 3. The American Red Cross estimates place the risk to be even lower, about 1 in 153,000.

97. Ibid.

98. John C. Petricciani and Jay S. Epstein, "The Effects of the AIDS Epidemic on the Safety of the Nation's Blood Supply," *Public Health Reports*, vol. 103 (May–June 1988), p. 240.

99. Richard J. Newman and Doug Podolsky with Penny Loeb, "Bad Blood," *U.S. News and World Report*, June 27, 1994, pp. 68–78.

100. Ibid.

101. Newman and Podolsky with Loeb, "Bad Blood."

102. For an elaboration on OSHA politics, see Foreman, *Signals from the Hill*, pp. 54–65, 108–14.

103. *Oversight Hearings on OSHA's Proposed Standard to Protect Health Care Workers against Blood-Borne Pathogens Including the AIDS and Hepatitis B Viruses— Volume 1*, Hearings before the Subcommittee on Health and Safety of the House Committee on Education and Labor, 101 Cong. 1 sess. (GPO, 1990), p. 178.

104. 54 Fed. Reg. 23134 (1989).

105. Ibid., p. 23135.

106. Steven Kelman, "Occupational Safety and Health Administration," in Wilson, *Politics of Regulation*, pp. 236–66.

107. *Oversight*, Hearings, pp. 33–34. For the CDC's November 15, 1985, recommendations on preventing HIV transmission in the workplace, see *Reports on AIDS*, pp. 128–35.

108. 54 Fed. Reg. 23047 (1989).

109. *Oversight*, Hearings, p. 238.

110. *Oversight of the Occupational Safety and Health Administration*, Hearings before the Senate Committee on Labor and Human Resources, 100 Cong. 2 sess. (GPO, 1988). More generally, see Foreman, "Legislators, Regulators, and the OMB," pp. 123–43.

111. Quoted at 56 Fed. Reg. 64092 (1991).

112. Ibid., p. 64093.

113. *Oversight*, Hearings, pp. 42–43.

114. Frank Swoboda, "OSHA Mandates AIDS Protection," *Washington Post*, December 3, 1991, pp. A1, A4. See also 56 Fed. Reg. 64004-182 (1991).

115. 56 Fed. Reg. 64175 (1991).

116. Ibid., pp. 64175, 64179.

117. M. J. Alter and others, "The Changing Epidemiology of Hepatitis B in the United States," *Journal of the American Medical Association*, March 2, 1990, pp. 1218–22.

118. This is why, despite some evidence of carcinogenicity and a clear statutory mandate indicating a ban, the FDA was expressly forbidden to withdraw saccharin from the market. Nor was the agency permitted to move quickly to reduce the heavy reliance of farmers on cattle and poultry feed laced with antibiotics, a practice associated with enhanced growth, higher profits, and the possible proliferation of drug-resistant microbes. See Foreman, *Signals from the Hill*, pp. 99–100, 137–41.

119. National Vaccine Information Center, *NVIC News* (Vienna, Va.: Dissatisfied Parents Together). Emphasis added.

120. David Vogel, "AIDS and the Politics of Drug Lag."

121. Malcolm Gladwell, "Beyond HIV: The Legacies of Health Activism," *Washington Post*, October 15, 1992, p. A29.

122. See *Congressional Record*, daily ed., October 7, 1992, pp. S17234–40.

123. See statement of Senator Edward M. Kennedy, Democrat of Massachusetts, at ibid., p. S17238. See also Malcolm Gladwell, "Congress Approves Measure to Speed FDA Drug Approval," *Washington Post*, October 8, 1992, pp. A1, A9.

Chapter Seven

1. General Accounting Office, *FDA's Oversight of the 1982 Canned Salmon Recalls*, GAO/HRD-84-77 (Washington, September 1984).

2. See Christopher H. Foreman, Jr., "Grassroots Victim Organizations: Mobilizing for Personal and Public Health," in Allan J. Cigler and Burdett Loomis, eds., *Interest Group Politics*, 4th ed. (Washington: Congressional Quarterly Press, forthcoming).

3. National Institutes of Health, *NIH Data Book—1993* (Bethesda, Md.: 1994), pp. 10, 13; and *Departments of Labor, Health and Human Services, Education, and Related Agencies Appropriations for 1993, Part 3, National Institutes of Health*, Hearings before the House Committee on Appropriations, 102 Cong. 2 sess. (Government Printing Office, 1992), pp. 22–23.

4. A discussion of such earmarking is Daryl E. Chubin and Edward J. Hackett, *Peerless Science: Peer Review and U.S. Science Policy* (State University of New York Press, 1990), pp. 153–62.

5. NIH, *NIH Data Book—1993*, p. 3.

6. The Federal Grant and Cooperative Agreement Act of 1977 (92 Stat. 4-5) distinguishes among the three in the following way. A grant is appropriate when "the principal purpose of the relationship is the transfer of [resources] . . . to accomplish a public purpose of support or stimulation authorized by Federal statute." A contract is the preferred mechanism when "the principal purpose . . . is the acquisition . . . of property or services for the direct benefit or use of the Federal Government." A cooperative agreement may be thought of as having the same purpose as a grant, except that "substantial involvement is anticipated between the executive agency . . . and the . . . recipient during performance of the contemplated activity."

7. NIH, *NIH Data Book—1993*, p. 31.

8. In formal NIH parlance, the term *review committee* generally refers to those first-stage peer review units operating under the auspices of the individual institutes. The term *study section* often is used in the same context. Strictly speaking, however, it applies only to the corresponding structures working for the Division of Research Grants. *Initial review group* is the preferred generic term referring to review committees and study sections equally.

9. National Cancer Act of 1971 (85 Stat. 778).

10. Presidential Commission on the Human Immunodeficiency Virus Epidemic, *Report of the Presidential Commission on the Human Immunodeficiency Virus Epidemic* (GPO, 1988), p. 38.

11. Robert Gallo, *Virus Hunting—AIDS, Cancer, and the Human Retrovirus: A Story of Scientific Discovery* (Basic Books, 1991), p. 139, and more generally chaps. 8–11. A retrovirus, unlike other viruses, carries a special enzyme called reverse transcriptase, allowing for the conversion of RNA to DNA, a peculiar stage in viral replication and the opposite of the usual DNA to RNA scenario.

12. See the *HHS News*, press release, Department of Health and Human Services, September 20, 1982. The very fact that grants totaling $165,195, an unremarkable sum, were deemed worthy of a press release suggests recognition of growing interest in, and perhaps defensiveness about, the disease.

13. Letter from Anthony S. Fauci, director, National Institute of Allergy and Infectious Diseases, to the author, April 2, 1991.

14. *AIDS Drugs: Where Are They?*, H. Rept. 100-1092, 100 Cong. 2 sess. (GPO, 1988), p. 3; and *The Federal Response to AIDS*, Hearings before the Subcommittee on Intergovernmental Relations and Human Resources of the House Committee on Government Operations, 98 Cong. 1 sess. (GPO, 1983), pp. 22–23.

15. Gina Kolata, "Congress, NIH Open Coffers for AIDS," in Ruth Kulstad, ed., *AIDS: Papers from Science, 1982–1985* (Washington: American Association for the Advancement of Science, 1986), p. 59.

16. *AIDS Research Act of 1988*, H. Rept. 100-815, 100 Cong. 2 sess. (GPO, 1988), p. 17.

17. *Report of the Presidential Commission*, p. 46.

18. Interview with an NIH official, July 26, 1990.

19. On rare occasions, slight delays may result from the complexity and cost of projects. One example was an RFP "for a multimillion dollar NIAID contract providing central data coordination for many different research studies

of AIDS treatment in over 30 clinical centers throughout the U.S." Another was a "multifaceted clinical study involving AIDS pathogenesis" with multiple awards anticipated and "coordinated with other similar projects in the awarding unit, NHLBI [the National Heart, Lung, and Blood Institute]." Both instances "involved complex evaluations of many factors, including site visits and other special review-award procedures." See NIH, "Implementation of AIDS Expedited Reviews and Awards—Report to the Congress," unpublished draft, obtained from files, NIH, Bethesda, Md., November 18, 1988, revised December 29, 1988, pp. 7–8.

20. See Department of Health and Human Services, Instruction and Information Memorandum OER-5 on triage of applications from the associate director for extramural affairs, obtained from files, NIH, Bethesda, Md., November 15, 1988.

21. Institute of Medicine, *Report of a Study: The AIDS Research Program of the National Institutes of Health* (Washington: National Academy Press, 1991), p. 37.

22. The data derive from the NIH database known as CRISP (Computer Retrieval of Information on Scientific Projects). For most grants, CRISP offers the names and addresses of principal investigators, abstracts of research projects (though not subprojects), and extramural funding amounts per fiscal year. It also classifies each project as either primary or secondary according to how strongly a given project is related to a particular ailment that is the subject of a search. Despite the many ambiguities that can bedevil any discussion based on such data, CRISP is nonetheless useful for roughly gauging the size and character of the focused NIH commitment to extramural research on particular diseases. All computations of dollar figures in the present discussion are for primary relationships only. See Sandra Panem, *The Interferon Crusade* (Brookings, 1984), pp. 38–41.

23. The funding of this epidemiologic study by the NIH exemplifies the sometimes imprecise division of labor between the NIH and the CDC. While the former is generally identified with basic bench science and the latter with epidemiologic investigation, agency turfs are not mutually exclusive in any absolute sense.

24. *Departments of Health and Human Services, Education, and Related Agencies Appropriations for 1992*, Hearings before the Subcommittee on the Departments of Labor, Health and Human Services, Education, and Related Agencies of the House Committee on Appropriations, 102 Cong. 1 sess. (GPO, 1991), p. 107. Figures include total obligations for all NIH components.

25. Michael Fumento, *The Myth of Heterosexual AIDS* (Basic Books, 1990); and Charles Krauthammer, "AIDS Hysteria," *New Republic*, October 5, 1987, p. 18.

26. Ron Brookmeyer, "Reconstruction and Future Trends of the AIDS Epidemic in the United States," *Science*, July 5, 1991, pp. 37–42.

27. Fumento, *The Myth*, p. 327.

28. A detailed activist critique of NIH AIDS research complains that "in 1990 Congress earmarked $40M for research on children with AIDS, especially

for clinical trials. Since there was no new money appropriated for this purpose the funds came directly from the adult AIDS Clinical Trials Group (ACTG). The result is that now, in 1992, the U.S. Government is spending $105.00 [on pediatric AIDS] research [for] every child with AIDS in America, compared with just $1.00 for each adult." See Gregg Gonsalves and Mark Harrington, *AIDS Research at the NIH: A Critical Review—Part 1: Summary* (New York: Treatment Action Group, 1992), p. 2.

29. Institute of Medicine, *Report of a Study*, p. 19.

30. Some individuals testing positive for HIV have continued to survive for many years with little or no resulting disease. Scientists and activists are desperate to learn why.

31. "Dying for Dollars," *New Republic*, December 17, 1990, pp. 7–8.

32. National Institute of Medicine, *Report of a Study*, pp. 23–24. By 1987 AIDS ranked fifteenth among causes of adult mortality in the United States. But by 1988 AIDS ranked sixth in years of potential life lost before age sixty-five.

33. Charles Backstrom and Leonard Robins, *The Minnesota Response to AIDS* (University of Minnesota, Center for Urban and Regional Affairs, 1992), p. 2.

34. J. Peter Nixon, "Budgeting during a Public Health Crisis: AIDS Budgeting at the National Institutes of Health," Georgetown University, May 1991.

35. Nixon, "Budgeting," pp. 15–16. On the concept of an annual incremental fair share as an aid to calculation in congressional appropriations decisionmaking, see Aaron B. Wildavsky, *The Politics of the Budgetary Process* (Little, Brown, 1964).

36. Stephen Burd, "Priorities for AIDS Research," *Chronicle of Higher Education*, January 5, 1994, p. A36.

37. "RML Scientists Discover the Cause of Lyme Disease," draft press release, National Institute for Allergies and Infectious Diseases, Bethesda, Md., June 1982, p. 2.

38. Peter S. Arno and Karyn L. Feiden, *Against the Odds: The Story of AIDS Drug Development, Politics, and Profits* (HarperCollins, 1992), pp. 192–93. See also *Drugs for Opportunistic Infections in Persons with HIV Disease*, Hearing before the Subcommittee on Human Resources and Intergovernmental Relations of the House Committee on Government Operations, 101 Cong. 2 sess. (GPO, 1991), p. 17.

39. *Departments of Labor, Health and Human Services, Education, and Related Agencies Appropriations for 1993: Part 3*, Hearings before the Subcommittee on the Departments of Labor, Health and Human Services, Education, and Related Agencies of the House Committee on Appropriations, 102 Cong. 2 sess. (GPO, 1992), p. 1153.

40. Joseph Palca, "On the Track of an Elusive Disease," *Science*, December 20, 1991, p. 1726.

41. Data from Tufts University Center for the Study of Drug Development, cited in Vance C. Gordon and Dale E. Wierenga, "The Drug Development and Approval Process," in "New Drug Approvals in 1990," press release, Pharmaceutical Manufacturers Association, Washington, D.C., January 1991.

42. Jon Cohen, "Did Liability Block AIDS Trial?" *Science*, July 17, 1992, pp. 316–17.

43. Jon Cohen, "Is Liability Slowing AIDS Vaccines?" *Science*, April 10, 1992, pp. 168–70.

44. Richard E. Neustadt and Harvey V. Fineberg, *The Epidemic That Never Was: Policy-Making and the Swine Flu Scare* (Vintage Books, 1983), chap. 7. See also Louis Lasagna, "The Chilling Effect of Product Liability on New Drug Development," in Peter W. Huber and Robert E. Litan, eds., *The Liability Maze: The Impact of Liability Law on Safety and Innovation* (Brookings, 1991), chap. 9.

45. See generally Arno and Feiden, *Against the Odds*, pp. 334–59; and Bruce Nussbaum, *Good Intentions: How Big Business and the Medical Establishment Are Corrupting the Fight against AIDS* (Atlantic Monthly Press, 1990).

46. Regarding unethical treatment of subjects, the infamous Tuskegee syphilis study comes to mind. See James H. Jones, *Bad Blood: The Tuskegee Syphilis Experiment* (Free Press, 1993). Marcel C. La Follette, *Stealing into Print: Fraud, Plagiarism, and Misconduct in Scientific Publishing* (University of California Press, 1992).

47. See Arno and Feiden, *Against the Odds*, chaps. 15, 17. See also Michael Specter, "AIDS Patients Insist on Treatment Role," *Washington Post*, June 5, 1989, p. A12; and Malcolm Gladwell, "Compound Q Debated at AIDS Forum," *Washington Post*, June 23, 1990, p. A8.

48. Marcia Barinaga, "Furor at Lyme Disease Conference," *Science*, June 5, 1992, pp. 1384–85.

49. See the comments of Barry R. Bloom, professor of microbiology and immunology at the Albert Einstein College of Medicine, in Rick Weiss, "On the Track of 'Killer' TB," *Science*, January 10, 1992, p. 148; and in Allan Freedman, "The Fall and Rise of Tuberculosis," *Government Executive*, vol. 24 (July 1992), pp. 14–16, 18.

50. A comprehensive and politically astute account of vaccine creation is Jane S. Smith, *Patenting the Sun: Polio and the Salk Vaccine* (Doubleday, 1990).

51. Human diseases for which vaccines are available include polio, measles, mumps, rubella (German measles), diphtheria, pertussis (whooping cough), tetanus, hepatitis B, *Haemophilus influenzae* B, rabies, yellow fever, plague, chicken pox, influenza, tuberculosis, cholera, smallpox, anthrax, adenovirus, and both pneumococcal and meningococcal disease. For a comprehensive review of the variety of vaccines, see Centers for Disease Control, "General Recommendations on Immunization," *Morbidity and Mortality Weekly Report*, Atlanta, January 28, 1994, p. 4. (Hereafter CDC, *MMWR*.) An engrossing treatment of Jenner is Peter Radetsky, *The Invisible Invaders: The Story of the Emerging Age of Viruses* (Little, Brown, and Company, 1991), pp. 25–37.

52. Abram S. Berenson, ed., *Control of Communicable Diseases in Man* (Washington: American Public Health Association, 1985), p. 195.

53. *Childhood Immunizations*, Hearing before the Subcommittee on Health and the Environment of the House Committee on Energy and Commerce, 101 Cong. 1 sess. (GPO, 1989), p. 52; and Don Colburn, "Measles Redux," *Washington Post*, September 1, 1992, p. 27. The CDC reported that some 20 percent of

reported measles cases in the United States in 1991 involved "appropriately vaccinated" individuals. See CDC, "Measles Summaries—United States, 1991," *MMWR*, November 20, 1992, p. 7.

54. Lawrence K. Altman, "Stymied by Resurgence of TB, Doctors Reconsider a Decades-Old Vaccine," *New York Times*, October 15, 1992, p. B4. See also Lawrence K. Altman, Tuberculosis Vaccine Found Surprisingly Effective in Study," *New York Times*, March 2, 1994, p. C14.

55. Institute of Medicine, *Vaccine Supply and Innovation* (Washington: National Academy Press, 1985), pp. 20–21.

56. A comprehensive review of the hurdles impeding the search for AIDS vaccines and therapies is "AIDS: The Unanswered Questions," *Science*, May 28, 1993, pp. 1254–93.

57. Erol Fikrig and others, "Protection of Mice against the Lyme Disease Agent by Immunizing with Recombinant OspA," *Science*, October 26, 1990, pp. 553–55.

58. R. Weiss, "Bio-tick-nology Yields Lyme Disease Vaccine," *Science News*, October 27, 1990, p. 261.

59. John Travis, "Biting Back at Lyme Disease," *Science*, June 19, 1992, p. 1623.

60. Weiss, "Bio-tick-nology."

61. Elisabeth Rosenthal, "Doctors Pin Hopes on Vaccine for Lyme," *New York Times*, September 21, 1993, pp. C1, C3.

62. Peter Radetsky, "Closing In on an AIDS Vaccine," *Discover*, vol. 11 (September 1990), pp. 70–77.

63. Joseph Palca, "Chimps Protected from Infected Cells," *Science*, June 19, 1992, p. 1632.

64. See Michael B. Agy and others, "Infection of *Macaca nemestrina* by Human Immunodeficiency Virus Type-1," *Science*, July 3, 1992, pp. 103–06; and Joseph Palca, "A Surprise Animal Model for AIDS," *Science*, June 19, 1992, pp. 1630–31.

65. Steve Sternberg, "HIV Comes in Five Family Groups," *Science*, May 15, 1992, p. 966.

66. An informed speculation that variation in viral genes may not pose insurmountable problems is Jon Cohen, "How Can Viral Variation Be Overcome?" *Science*, May 28, 1993, p. 1260.

67. Malcolm Gladwell, "AIDS Vaccine Test Yields Cautious Hope," *Washington Post*, December 18, 1992, pp. A1, A27. The findings are available in Muthiah D. Daniel and others, "Protective Effects of a Live Attenuated SIV Vaccine with a Deletion in the *nef* Gene," *Science*, December 18, 1992, pp. 1938–41.

68. Jon Cohen, "Jitters Jeopardize AIDS Vaccine Trials," *Science*, November 12, 1993, pp. 980–81, and "A New Goal: Preventing Disease, Not Infection," *Science*, December 17, 1993, pp. 1820–21.

69. Christopher P. Howson, Cynthia J. Howe, and Harvey V. Fineberg, eds., *Adverse Effects of Pertussis and Rubella Vaccines: A Report of the Committee to Review the Adverse Consequences of Pertussis and Rubella Vaccines* (Washington: National Academy Press, 1991), p. 17.

70. See, for example, the various case histories distributed throughout Harris L. Cloulter and Barbara Loe Fisher, *A Shot in the Dark* (Avery Publishing Group, 1991).

71. CDC, "Pertussis Vaccination: Acellular Pertussis Vaccine for Reinforcing and Booster Use—Supplementary ACIP Statement," *MMWR*, February 7, 1992, p. 3.

72. "Vaccine for Whooping Cough Is Approved by Government," *New York Times*, December 19, 1991, p. B22.

73. An example of a new pathogen that proved self-limiting in most cases was *Legionella*. The overwhelming majority of victims recover even without specific treatment.

74. Arno and Feiden, *Against the Odds.*

75. *AIDS Treatment Research and Approval*, Hearing before the Senate Committee on Labor and Human Resources, 100 Cong. 2 sess. (GPO, 1988), p. 158.

76. Joshua Lederberg, Robert E. Shope, and Stanley C. Oaks, Jr., eds., *Emerging Infections: Microbial Threats to Health in the United States* (Washington: National Academy Press, 1992), pp. 98–99.

77. Allen C. Steere, "Lyme Disease," *New England Journal of Medicine*, August 31, 1989, pp. 586–96.

78. John J. Halperin, David J. Volkman, and Priscilla Wu, "Central Nervous System Abnormalities in Lyme Neuroborreliosis," *Neurology*, vol. 41 (October 1991), pp. 1571–81.

79. Brian R. Edlin and others, "An Outbreak of Multidrug-Resistant Tuberculosis among Hospitalized Patients with the Acquired Immunodeficiency Syndrome," *New England Journal of Medicine*, June 4, 1992, p. 1520.

80. Susan Okie, "NIH Creates High-Level AIDS Post," *Washington Post*, May 3, 1988, p. A25.

81. National Institute of Allergy and Infectious Diseases, *ACTG in Depth* (Bethesda, Md.: NIH, May 1990).

82. Aerosolized pentamidine is used to inhibit *Pneumocystis carinii* pneumonia in persons with HIV disease. For a detailed critical history of government activity leading up to its approval as an AIDS treatment, see Arno and Feiden, *Against the Odds*, chap. 8.

83. See Thomas C. Merigan, "You *Can* Teach an Old Dog New Tricks," *New England Journal of Medicine*, November 8, 1990, pp. 1341–43; and David P. Byar and others, "Design Considerations for AIDS Trials," *New England Journal of Medicine*, November 8, 1990, pp. 1343–48.

84. See Public Law 101-381, sec. 2671 (104 Stat. 617).

85. Telephone interview with Tom Forschner, executive director, Lyme Disease Foundation, Tolland, Conn., September 11, 1992.

86. See Foreman, "Grassroots Victim Organizations."

87. "A Critique of the AIDS Clinical Trials Group" is reprinted in *Drugs for Opportunistic Infections*, Hearing, pp. 34–104. Quotation is on p. 43.

88. Ibid., p. 107.

89. Gonsalves and Harrington, *AIDS Research at the NIH*, pp. 4, 9.

90. Jon Cohen, "Task Force to Speed Drug Pipeline," *Science*, December 10, 1993, p. 1641.

91. Geoffrey Conley, "The Angry Politics of Kemron," *Newsweek*, January 4, 1993, pp. 43–44.

92. "Key Lobbyist Wins AIDS Vaccine Trials," *New York Times*, October 20, 1992, p. C2.

93. Barry Meier, "Scientists Assail Congress on Bill for Money to Test an AIDS Drug," *New York Times*, October 26, 1992, pp. A1, B8. In letters to Congress, the Department of Defense, the NIH, and the FDA killed the gp160 project by certifying that it should not go forward. Instead, the $20 million would go into a general fund for vaccine therapy research. Jon Cohen, "Peer Review Triumphs over Lobbying," *Science*, January 28, 1994, p. 463.

94. Gina Kolata, "AIDS Researchers Seek Redirection of Efforts toward Learning Basics of the Disease," *New York Times*, May 12, 1994, p. A20.

Chapter Eight

1. Joseph G. Morone and Edward J. Woodhouse, *Averting Catastrophe: Strategies for Regulating Risky Technologies* (University of California Press, 1986).

2. Howard M. Leichter, *Free to Be Foolish: Politics and Health Promotion in the United States and Great Britain* (Princeton University Press, 1991). Between 1965 and 1985 smoking prevalence "declined at a rate of 0.5 percentage points per year, and from 1987 through 1990 the rate of decline accelerated to 1.1 percentage points per year." As of 1991 some 46.3 million adults (25.7 percent) were "current smokers," defined as persons who reported a lifetime consumption of at least one hundred cigarettes and were currently smoking. These data are contained in Centers for Disease Control, *Morbidity and Mortality Weekly Report*, Atlanta, April 2, 1993, pp. 230–33. (Hereafter CDC, *MMWR*.)

3. Although genetic mutation complicates the problem of coping with dangerous microorganisms such as influenza and HIV, this factor is sometimes overemphasized. See Stephen S. Morse, "Examining the Origins of Emerging Viruses," in Morse, ed., *Emerging Viruses* (Oxford University Press, 1993), p. 12; and Stephen C. Joseph, *Dragon within the Gates: The Once and Future AIDS Epidemic* (Carroll and Graf, 1992), p. 48.

4. N. F. Stanley and R. A. Joske, eds., *Changing Disease Patterns and Human Behavior* (New York: Academic Press, 1980); Joshua Lederberg, Robert E. Shope, and Stanley C. Oaks, Jr., eds., *Emerging Infections: Microbial Threats to Health in the United States* (Washington: National Academy Press, 1992).

5. Elisabeth Rosenthal, "Outwitted by Malaria, Desperate Doctors Seek New Remedies," *New York Times*, February 12, 1991, pp. C1, C8; CDC, *MMWR*, August 30, 1991, pp. 585–91. On the measles epidemic of 1989–91, see "The Measles Menace," editorial, *New York Times*, February 21, 1991, p. A20; and CDC, "Measles—United States, 1992," *MMWR*, May 21, 1993, pp. 378–81. On the problem of antibiotic resistance, see Stuart B. Levy, *The Antibiotic Paradox: How Miracle Drugs Are Destroying the Miracle* (Plenum Press, 1992).

6. Aaron Wildavsky, *Searching for Safety* (New Brunswick, N.J.: Transaction Books, 1988), chap. 3.

7. Ronald Bayer and others, "The Dual Epidemics of Tuberculosis and AIDS: Ethical and Policy Issues in Screening and Treatment," *American Journal of Public Health*, vol. 83 (May 1993), p. 652.

8. By the same token, modern cooling systems can facilitate the growth of *Legionella*. Polio outbreaks began only in the twentieth century as a paradoxical effect of increased sanitation. As one chronicler reported, "When people were no longer in contact with the open sewers and privies that had once exposed them to the polio virus in very early infancy, when paralysis rarely occurs, the disease changed from an endemic condition so mild that no one even knew it existed to a seemingly new epidemic threat of mysterious origins and terrifyingly unknown scope." Jane S. Smith, *Patenting the Sun: Polio and the Salk Vaccine* (Doubleday, 1990), p. 35.

9. Timothy Egan, "Tainted Hamburger Raises Doubts on Meat Safety," *New York Times*, January 27, 1993, p. A10; and Michael McCarthy, "Hamburger Hazard," *Washington Post*, February 9, 1993, pp. 8–10.

10. Eliot Marshall, "Hantavirus Outbreak Yields to PCR," *Science*, November 5, 1993, pp. 832–36.

11. Wildavsky, *Searching for Safety*, chap. 4.

12. Ibid., p. 77.

13. Ibid.

14. Michael deCourcy Hinds, "Survey Finds Flaws in States' Water Inspections," *New York Times*, April 15, 1993, p. A14. For an overview of the outbreak of cryptosporidiosis in Milwaukee, see J. Madeleine Nash, "The Waterworks Flu," *Time*, April 19, 1993, p. 41.

15. On the Cutter incident, see Smith, *Patenting the Sun*, pp. 359–70. On the drug law reforms, see Paul J. Quirk, "Food and Drug Administration," in James Q. Wilson, ed., *The Politics of Regulation* (Basic Books, 1980), pp. 195–97.

16. Agreement often cannot be reached on what knowing is. What constitutes acceptable or sufficient knowledge is also debated.

17. Sara Terry, "Drinking Water Comes to a Boil," *New York Times Magazine*, September 26, 1993, pp. 42–45, 48, 62, 65.

18. Randy Shilts, *And the Band Played On: Politics, People, and the AIDS Epidemic* (St. Martin's Press, 1987), pp. 18–20, 38–40.

19. Wolf Szmuness and others, "On the Role of Sexual Behavior in the Spread of Hepatitis B Infection," *Annals of Internal Medicine*, vol. 83 (October 1975), pp. 489–95; and M. T. Schreeder and others, "Hepatitis B in Homosexual Men: Prevalence of Infection and Factors Related to Transmission," *Journal of Infectious Diseases*, vol. 146 (July 1982), pp. 7–15.

20. As Baruch S. Blumberg, winner of the Nobel Prize for his elucidation of hepatitis B antigen, observed: "Many cases result in an acute disease which can be disabling but usually progresses to a complete recovery." See his "Hepatitis B Virus and the Carrier Problem," in Arien Mack, ed., *In Time of Plague: The History and Social Consequences of Lethal Epidemic Disease* (New York University Press, 1991), p. 80.

21. Milton Helpern, "Malaria among Drug Addicts in New York City," *Public Health Reports*, March 30, 1934, reprinted in *Public Health Reports*, vol. 91 (September–October 1976), pp. 477–79.

22. Stephen Barlay, *The Final Call: Why Airline Disasters Continue to Happen* (Pantheon Books, 1990), chap. 2.

23. Levy, *The Antibiotic Paradox*, chap. 6, pp. 137–56. See also Christopher H. Foreman, Jr., *Signals from the Hill: Congressional Oversight and the Challenge of Social Regulation* (Yale University Press, 1988), pp. 99–100.

24. Foreman, *Signals from the Hill*, pp. 137–41.

25. *FDA Issues*, Hearings before the Subcommittee on Health and the Environment of the House Committee on Energy and Commerce, 99 Cong. 1 sess. (Government Printing Office, 1985). See especially p. 127.

26. James Chin, "Raw Milk: A Continuing Vehicle for the Transmission of Infectious Disease Agents in the United States," *Journal of Infectious Diseases*, vol. 146 (September 1982), p. 440.

27. CDC, *Addressing Emerging Infectious Disease Threats: A Prevention Strategy for the United States*, (Atlanta, 1994), p. 2. This document defines an emerging infectious disease as one "of infectious origin whose incidence in humans has increased within the past two decades or threatens to increase in the near future" (p. 7). The term *emergent public health hazard* employed in this book is both narrower and broader. It includes only communicable diseases that have achieved some measure of recent media visibility but also embraces product hazards of which the same can be said.

28. Though unfortunately titled—heterosexual AIDS is no myth—a good source here is Michael Fumento, *The Myth of Heterosexual AIDS: How a Tragedy Has Been Distorted by the Media and Partisan Politics* (New Republic Books/Basic Books, 1990).

29. One might argue that the swine flu program represents anticipation rather than resilience. But given the senses in which Wildavsky employs these terms, I regard the latter as more appropriate. CDC Director David Sencer's recommendation was "anticipatory" in attempting to prevent a larger outbreak, but "resilient" in responding to evidence of a concrete (not merely hypothetical) hazard.

30. Richard E. Neustadt and Harvey V. Fineberg, *The Epidemic That Never Was: Policy-Making and the Swine Flu Scare* (Vintage Books, 1983). See also Stephen Fried, "Prescription for Disaster," *Washington Post Magazine*, April 3, 1994, pp. 12–16, 27–30.

31. Ibid., chaps. 12, 13; and Arthur M. Silverstein, *Pure Politics and Impure Science: The Swine Flu Affair* (Johns Hopkins University Press, 1981).

32. Ronald Bayer, *Private Acts, Social Consequences: AIDS and the Politics of Public Health* (Free Press, 1989), pp. 234–35; and Shilts, *And the Band Played On*, p. 533.

33. Operating room politics (high complexity, high salience) is characterized by intense participation and media scrutiny and results in laws and rules anchored in both professional norms and political considerations. Alternative situations are boardroom politics (high complexity, low salience), hearing room

politics (low complexity, high salience), and street-level politics (low complexity, low salience). See William T. Gormley, Jr., "Regulatory Issue Networks in a Federal System," *Polity*, vol. 18 (Summer 1986), pp. 595–620.

34. Joseph, *Dragon*, pp. 87–89.

35. Stuart L. Nightingale, "From the Food and Drug Administration," *Journal of the American Medical Association*, June 16, 1993, p. 2964.

36. Raymond L. Woosley, "A Prescription for Better Prescriptions," *Issues in Science and Technology*, vol. 10 (Spring 1994), pp. 59–66.

37. CDC, *Addressing Emerging Infectious Disease Threats*. For additional arguments for strengthened international surveillance to detect emerging microbial threats, see Stephen S. Morse, "Regulating Viral Traffic," *Issues in Science and Technology*, vol. 7 (Fall 1990), pp. 81–84; and Donald A. Henderson, "Surveillance Systems and Intergovernmental Cooperation," in Morse, *Emerging Viruses*, pp. 283–89.

38. According to the CDC proposal, "In 12 of the 50 states surveyed, no professional position is dedicated to surveillance of foodborne and waterborne diseases. Funding for communicable disease surveillance is largely confined to diseases for which public health crises have already developed; over 95% of funds allocated to states for infectious disease surveillance are targeted to four disease categories (TB, HIV/AIDS, sexually transmitted diseases . . . and selected vaccine preventable diseases) with no federal resources going to state and local health agencies to sustain the national notifiable disease system." CDC, *Addressing Emerging Infectious Disease Threats*, p. 3.

39. Edwin D. Kilbourne, letter to *Issues in Science and Technology*, vol. 7 (Spring 1991), p. 22.

40. P.L. 98-49.

41. *Health and the Environment: Miscellaneous—Part 1*, Hearings before the Subcommittee on Health and the Environment of the House Committee on Energy and Commerce, 98 Cong. 1 sess. (GPO, 1983).

42. Peter S. Arno and Karyn Feiden, "Ignoring the Epidemic: How the Reagan Administration Failed on AIDS," *Health PAC Bulletin*, vol. 17 (December 1986), p. 9.

43. *Agriculture, Rural Development, Food and Drug Administration, and Related Appropriations for 1993*, Hearings before the Subcommittee on Agriculture, Rural Development, Food and Drug Administration, and Related Agencies of the House Committee on Appropriations, 102 Cong. 2 sess. (GPO, 1992), p. 49.

44. See, for example, the NIH appropriations for 1994 contained in P.L. 103-112.

45. *Departments of Labor, Health and Human Services, Education, and Related Agencies Appropriations for 1993—Part 3, National Institutes of Health*, Hearings before the Subcommittee on the Departments of Labor, Health and Human Services, Education, and Related Agencies of the House Committee on Appropriations, 102 Cong. 2 sess. (GPO, 1992), pp. 4, 148.

46. As the CDC's *Addressing Emerging Infectious Disease Threats* noted: "To rapidly and effectively address the outbreak of Hantavirus Pulmonary Syndrome [in 1993], professional and support staff were reassigned for several

months—from other high priority programs. The availability of contingency funds for field investigations and the maintenance of adequate depth in person-nel infrastructure at CDC would help prevent such situations" (p. 19).

47. Quotation by Edward N. Brandt, Assistant Secretary for Health and Human Services, in *Health and the Environment, Miscellaneous—Part 1*, Hearing, p. 7.

48. Ibid., p. 50.

49. *Food, Drug, Cosmetic, and Device Enforcement Amendments*, Hearing before the Subcommittee on Health and the Environment of the House Committee on Energy and Commerce, 102 Cong. 1 sess. (GPO, 1991), p. 28.

50. Ibid., pp. 154–88.

51. Note, for example, Commissioner David Kessler's aggressive and suc-cessful campaign to unite Congress and the pharmaceutical industry behind a novel user-fee scheme to finance the increase of its drug evaluation and review staff by some six hundred positions. See Richard Stone, "FDA Sets Out to Hire 600—and Image Is a Problem," *Science*, November 6, 1992, p. 886. The most recent advisory overview of FDA performance also stresses resource constraints far more than cumbersome field enforcement. See Department of Health and Human Services, *Final Report of the Advisory Committee on the Food and Drug Administration* (Washington, May 1991).

52. The NIH Revitalization Act of 1993 (P.L. 103-43, sec. 1801) created an office of AIDS research to plan and coordinate all AIDS-related research activi-ties in the agency. The director of the office has access to a substantial emergency discretionary fund authorized to grow as high as $100 million. This is not a broad contingency fund because the OAR director's money is devoted solely to AIDS. A number of additional legislative preconditions and limitations govern the fund's use.

53. *America Living with AIDS*, Report of the National Commission on Acquired Immune Deficiency Syndrome (Washington: National Commission on the Acquired Immune Deficiency Syndrome, 1991), p. 120.

54. Ibid. A similar proposal is offered in Sandra Panem, *The AIDS Bureau-cracy: Why Society Failed to Meet the AIDS Crisis and How We Might Improve Our Response* (Harvard University Press, 1988), chap. 10.

55. Jon Cohen, "A 'Manhattan Project' for AIDS?" *Science*, February 19, 1993, pp. 1112–14. See also Larry Kramer, "A 'Manhattan Project' for AIDS," *New York Times*, July 16, 1990, p. A15.

56. Christopher H. Foreman, Jr., "AIDS and the Limits of Czardom: Why We Can't 'Coordinate' an End to the Epidemic," *Brookings Review*, vol. 11 (Summer 1993), pp. 18–21.

57. Richard Rhodes, *The Making of the Atomic Bomb* (Simon and Schuster, 1988). On the state of scientific knowledge regarding AIDS, see the various essays in *Science*, May 28, 1993.

58. Giuseppe Pantaleo, Cecilia Graziosi, and Anthony S. Fauci, "The Immu-nopathogenesis of Human Immunodeficiency Virus Infection," *New England Journal of Medicine*, February 4, 1993, pp. 327, 333.

59. Amy Goldstein, "Clean Needle Programs for Addicts Proliferate," *Washington Post*, April 23, 1991, p. 6. See also David L. Kirp and Ronald Bayer, "Public Health: Needles and Race," *Atlantic Monthly*, vol. 272 (July 1993), pp. 38–39, 42. GAO, *Needle Exchange Programs: Research Suggests Promise as an AIDS Prevention Strategy*, GAO/HRD-93-60 (Washington, March 1993). Stephen B. Thomas and Sandra Crouse Quinn, "The Burdens of Race and History on Black Attitudes toward Needle Exchange Policy to Prevent HIV Disease," *Journal of Public Health Policy*, vol. 13 (Autumn 1993), pp. 320–47.

60. Harvey M. Sapolsky, *The Polaris System Development: Bureaucratic and Programmatic Success in Government* (Harvard University Press, 1972).

61. Charles Perrow and Mauro F. Guillén, *The AIDS Disaster: The Failure of Organizations in New York and the Nation* (Yale University Press, 1990), pp. 181–83.

62. Ibid., pp. 182–83.

63. Albert R. Jonsen and Jeff Stryker, eds., *The Social Impact of AIDS in the United States* (Washington: National Academy Press, 1993).

64. Consider, for example, the fate of AIDS test developer Mika Popovic, who lost his job at the NIH for relatively small mistakes on the road to doing "one incomparably great thing." See Malcolm Gladwell, "Science Friction," *Washington Post Magazine*, December 6, 1992, pp. 18–21, 49–51.

65. Gina Kolata, "Targeting Urged in Attack on AIDS," *New York Times*, March 7, 1993, p. 1.

66. See "HIV Prevention: An Update on the Status of Methods Women Can Use," and "'Getting Real' about HIV and Homeless Youth," *American Journal of Public Health*, October 1, 1993, pp. 1379, 1490.

67. Perrow and Guillén, *The AIDS Disaster*, pp. 18–19.

68. On this point, see H. Jack Geiger, "Plenty of Blame to Go Around," *New York Times Book Review*, November 8, 1987, p. 9.

Index